Physical Medicine and Rehabilitation
Oral Board Review

Physical Medicine and Rehabilitation Oral Board Review

Interactive Case Discussions

Editor

R. Samuel Mayer, MD, MEHP
Associate Professor and Vice Chair, Education
Department of Physical Medicine and Rehabilitation
Johns Hopkins University School of Medicine
Baltimore, Maryland

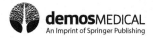
demosMEDICAL
An Imprint of Springer Publishing

Visit our website at www.demosmedical.com

ISBN: 9781620701072
ebook ISBN: 9781617052859

Acquisitions Editor: Beth Barry
Compositor: Diacritech

Medicine is an ever-changing science. Research and clinical experience are continually expanding our knowledge, in particular our understanding of proper treatment and drug therapy. The authors, editors, and publisher have made every effort to ensure that all information in this book is in accordance with the state of knowledge at the time of production of the book. Nevertheless, the authors, editors, and publisher are not responsible for errors or omissions or for any consequences from application of the information in this book and make no warranty, expressed or implied, with respect to the contents of the publication. Every reader should examine carefully the package inserts accompanying each drug and should carefully check whether the dosage schedules mentioned therein or the contraindications stated by the manufacturer differ from the statements made in this book. Such examination is particularly important with drugs that are either rarely used or have been newly released on the market.

Library of Congress Cataloging-in-Publication Data
Names: Mayer, R. Samuel, editor.
Title: Physical medicine and rehabilitation oral board review : interactive
  case discussions / [edited by] R. Samuel Mayer.
Description: New York : Demos Medical Publishing, [2018] | Includes
  bibliographical references and index.
Identifiers: LCCN 2017032271| ISBN 9781620701072 | ISBN 9781617052859 (e-book)
Subjects: | MESH: Physical Therapy Modalities | Rehabilitation—methods |
  Examination Questions | Case Reports
Classification: LCC RM701.6 | NLM WB 18.2 | DDC 615.8/2076—dc23 LC record available at
  https://lccn.loc.gov/2017032271

Printed in the United States of America by Gasch Printing.
17 18 19 20 21 / 5 4 3 2 1

Contents

Contributors

Matthew N. Bartels, MD
Professor and Chair
The Arthur S. Abramson Department of Physical Medicine and Rehabilitation
Montefiore Medical Center
Bronx, New York

Bryt Christensen, MD, FABPMR
Interventional Pain Physician
Southwest Spine and Pain Center
St. George, Utah

Tae Chung, MD
Assistant Professor
Department of Physical Medicine and Rehabilitation
Johns Hopkins University School of Medicine
Baltimore, Maryland

Brad E. Dicianno, MD
Associate Professor
Department of Physical Medicine and Rehabilitation
University of Pittsburgh School of Medicine
Pittsburgh, Pennsylvania

George Forrest, MD
Department of Rehabilitation Medicine
Albany Medical College
Albany, New York

Stephen Johnson, MD
Clinical Assistant Professor
Department of Rehabilitation Medicine
University of Washington
Seattle, Washington

Sarah Korth, MD
Attending Physician, Kennedy Krieger Institute
Assistant Professor
Department of Physical Medicine and Rehabilitation
Johns Hopkins University School of Medicine
Baltimore, Maryland

Brian J. Krabak, MD, MBA, FACSM
Clinical Professor
Rehabilitation, Orthopedics and Sports Medicine
University of Washington and Seattle Children's Hospital
Seattle, Washington

Brian C. Liem, MD
Clinical Assistant Professor
Department of Rehabilitation Medicine
University of Washington
Seattle, Washington

Melinda S. Loveless, MD
Clinical Assistant Professor
Department of Rehabilitation Medicine
University of Washington
Seattle, Washington

Michael Mallow, MD
Assistant Professor
Department of Rehabilitation Medicine
Sidney Kimmel Medical College at Thomas Jefferson University
Philadelphia, Pennsylvania

Michael H. Marino, MD
Attending Physician
MossRehab, Einstein Healthcare Network
Elkins Park, Pennsylvania

R. Samuel Mayer, MD, MEHP
Associate Professor and Vice Chair, Education
Department of Physical Medicine and Rehabilitation
Johns Hopkins University School of Medicine
Baltimore, Maryland

Nathan Neufeld, DO
Medical Director of Pain Services and Supportive Therapies and Interventional
    Pain Management Specialist
Southeastern Regional Medical Center
Newnan, Georgia

Frank Pidcock, MD
Vice President, Department of Rehabilitation at Kennedy Krieger Institute
Director, Pediatric Rehabilitation Division, Department of Physical Medicine
    and Rehabilitation
Johns Hopkins Hospital and University School of Medicine
Associate Professor of Physical Medicine and Rehabilitation and Associate
    Professor of Pediatrics
Johns Hopkins University School of Medicine
Baltimore, Maryland

Miriam Segal, MD
Attending Physician
MossRehab, Einstein Healthcare Network
Elkins Park, Pennsylvania

Julie K. Silver, MD
Associate Professor/Associate Chair and Director of Cancer Rehabilitation
Department of Physical Medicine and Rehabilitation
Harvard Medical School/Spaulding Rehabilitation Network
Boston, Massachusetts

Argyrios Stampas, MD
SCI Medicine Research Director/Assistant Professor
Department of Physical Medicine and Rehabilitation
UTHealth Science Center
Houston, Texas

J. George Thomas, MD
Physical Medicine and Rehabilitation
Carolinas HealthCare System Rehabilitation
Charlotte, North Carolina

Melissa Trovato, MD
Director of Inpatient Rehabilitation
Kennedy Krieger Institute
Assistant Professor
Department of Physical Medicine and Rehabilitation
Johns Hopkins School of Medicine
Baltimore, Maryland

Heikki Uustal, MD
Associate Professor
Physical Medicine and Rehabilitation
Rutgers-Robert Wood Johnson Medical School
Piscataway, New Jersey

Thomas Watanabe, MD
Clinical Director
Drucker Brain Injury Center
MossRehab, Einstein Healthcare Network
Elkins Park, Pennsylvania

Introduction

R. Samuel Mayer

Physical medicine and rehabilitation (PM&R) is one of the broadest and most challenging specialties in medicine. Physiatrists see patients of all age groups with impairments of every organ system, and must have keen understanding of anatomy, biomechanics, ergonomics, exercise physiology, kinesiology, neurophysiology, pharmacology, and psychology. They not only prescribe medications and perform procedures, but also prescribe prosthetics, orthotics, splints, and complex medical equipment. They lead interdisciplinary teams that address the holistic bio-psycho-social and spiritual needs of people with disabling conditions. No wonder board certification preparation becomes a daunting task for examinees.

ABOUT THE EXAM

In PM&R, board certification has three components: Part I is a written examination, testing medical knowledge; Part II is an oral examination that tests clinical practice skills. The third component is maintenance of certification (MOC), which is an ongoing educational and evaluation process after attainment of initial certification. Part I is taken in August after completion of residency training. Nine months later (in May), examinees can take Part II, after passing Part I and gaining some experience in clinical practice or fellowship. The final component is ongoing MOC, which promotes lifelong learning.

The Part I exam focuses on knowledge. The knowledge base for PM&R has enormous breadth and depth. However, the process of studying for a knowledge-based test should be familiar to most physicians. There are a host of textbooks, several board review books, and a number of question banks available to hone one's familiarity with the field.

Part II, on the other hand, tests skills and behaviors. The Accreditation Committee for Graduate Medical Education (ACGME) defined six core competencies for physicians: medical knowledge, clinical care, practice-based learning, communication, professionalism, and systems-based practice. Part I tests the first of these competencies, while Part II tests the remainder. How does one study for this?

I would first advise that "studying" is the wrong approach. One attains skills by doing, not by reading about them. It takes practice, practice, practice. You will learn most from your patients; listen to them carefully as their stories will enlighten you. Next, take advantage of your mentors' skills and experience. Watch them examine patients, scoop up their pearls, and, above all, ask them questions and get their feedback.

The case scenarios in this book are those encountered every day at the bedside. In general, the cases used by the American Board of Physical Medicine and Rehabilitation (ABPMR) are not exotic or esoteric; they are meant to cover common problems encountered in general physiatric practice. The emphasis is on clinical practice, not trivial pursuit of obscure medical knowledge. You will not be asked to recite the medical literature, although it can help you to use clinical guidelines in your answers to demonstrate familiarity with evidence-based medicine. Be specific but concise in your responses. Each examiner is given 40 minutes to review three to four cases with you. The cases are standardized. You do not need to complete all of the cases to pass. Often the last one or two cases that an examiner has to present are trial cases that the board is testing out for psychometric properties and not used in the actual scoring. You will have three examiners. The time schedule is rigid.

HOW TO USE THIS BOOK

This workbook is an additional tool, unique in its format. It walks the reader through cases in an interactive format. While it can be used individually, many may choose to use it with a partner or in small groups, so that learners can give answers aloud, simulating the oral board exam.

The cases are structured in a similar format to the ABPMR Part II. The content mirrors the exam outline, which is available on the ABPMR website. Although none of the authors are current oral examiners (this would be a conflict of interest), all are board certified and highly experienced clinicians, many with national and international reputations for excellence in their subspecialties.

The exam consists of questions about case vignettes. Each vignette fits into one or more diagnostic categories (there are nine broad diagnostic categories), and each may focus on one or more evaluation or management skills. Each case tests five clinical skills: data acquisition, problem solving, patient management, system-based practice, and interpersonal communication and professionalism. Each vignette in this book also has questions about each of these clinical skills.

We have used icons to code the questions to correspond to these five clinical skills:

 Data acquisition questions typically focus on the history and physical exam.

 Problem solving frequently deals with diagnostic skills or biomechanics.

 Patient management includes all aspects of treatment: medication, equipment, injections, rehabilitation therapies, and referrals to other specialists, including surgery.

 System-based practice refers to psychosocial and economic issues; quality improvement projects may also be discussed.

 Communication skills will be evaluated by the examiners. Be prepared to explain things in lay terms as if you were talking to a patient.

HINTS

Here are some hints for examinees. Dress and act professionally. Dress tends to be more formal than most clinical workplaces. Men wear suits and ties; women may also wear suits or conservative skirts and blouses. Treat these case vignettes like real patients; picture the examiner as a patient in front of you. Ask open-ended questions of the examiner; get additional detail on the patient's history and physical exam. Be empathetic and sensitive in your communication, just as you would be with a real patient. Be cautious not to violate ethical standards like patient privacy and informed consent in your answers. Speak slowly and articulate clearly. Use proper grammar. Do not be self-conscious if you have an accent—we all have accents of some type. Although easier said than done, be calm and natural, confident but not cocky.

While this text is intended as a board review workbook to be used in preparation for the Part II exam, other audiences will find it helpful as well. All PM&R residents and fellows should have a copy—it is never too early to prepare for the oral exam. Residency program directors and faculty will find these cases useful in bedside and didactic instruction. Those preparing for MOC should also find this useful. Practicing clinicians can use these vignettes to hone up on skills in patient populations that they see less frequently.

1 Amputee Care and Prosthetic Prescription

Heikki Uustal

CASE 1: BELOW KNEE AMPUTATION: DYSVASCULAR

A 72-year-old male with diabetes, neuropathy, and peripheral vascular disease presents with recent right below knee amputation (1 week ago) secondary to infection in the foot. Acute care physical therapy was able to mobilize the patient to wheelchair mobility and limited hopping 20 feet with a walker. His cardiovascular status is stable and the patient has only minimal pain, controlled with medications.

Questions

1. The patient is asking about his functional potential with a prosthesis. What further information regarding his history or previous activity will help to predict his functional outcome?

2. As you examine the patient, what are the three most critical muscle groups in the lower limb and the upper limb to prepare for prosthetic ambulation?

3. As you examine the residual limb, there are several important aspects to assess and document. List at least four of these.

4. The patient is now going to subacute rehabilitation or home with home therapy. What are the essential components of the pre-prosthetic program to prepare for prosthetic fitting?

5. As part of the process of prescribing a prosthesis, the ordering physician must establish and document the patient's "functional level" (also known as K-level) as defined by Medicare. The functional level will determine the category of prosthetic foot or knee allowed. Describe the functional levels.

6. Patient education and support during the pre-prosthetic and prosthetic phase are critical for patient understanding and participation. What issues in the psychosocial realm should be reviewed at each visit?

CASE 1: BELOW KNEE AMPUTATION: DYSVASCULAR

Answers

1. The patient's functional mobility status prior to amputation and the length of time since he last walked a significant distance are the two important factors to determine his potential for future ambulation with a prosthesis.

2. Lower limb: Hip extensors, knee extensors, hip abductors. Grade 4/5 strength in these muscles is critical to get from sit to stand and maintain stability during ambulation. Upper limb: Elbow extensors, shoulder depressors (pectoralis, latissimus). Grade 4/5 strength in these muscles is necessary to allow a patient to support himself or herself with an assistive device and prevent falls.

3. Bone length, soft tissue coverage, skin integrity, healing status of the surgical site, sensation, tenderness to palpation, shape of the residual limb, and soft tissue mobility.

4. The goals of pre-prosthetic physical therapy/occupational therapy programs include strengthening of the critical muscles, prevention of contractures (hips and knees), improvement in cardiopulmonary endurance to meet the additional demands of prosthetic use, progress in mobility, desensitizing the limb, shrinking and shaping of the residual limb, education, and home exercise program.

5. K-levels are:
   0 = nonambulatory
   1 = transfers or limited household ambulatory
   2 = household and limited community ambulatory
   3 = unlimited community ambulatory
   4 = high energy or activity beyond normal ambulation

6. Psychological adjustment to limb loss, evidence of depression, pain control, support/interaction with friends and family, and patient concerns about return to previous activity.

BIBLIOGRAPHY

Edelstein JE, Moroz A. *Lower-Limb Prosthetics and Orthotics: Clinical Concepts.* Thorofare, NJ: SLACK; 2011.

Esquenazi A. Amputation rehabilitation and prosthetic restoration. From surgery to community reintegration. *Disabil Rehabil.* 2004;26:831-836.

Smith DG, Michael JW, Bowker JH. *Atlas of Amputations and Limb Deficiencies: Surgical, Prosthetic, and Rehabilitation Principles.* 3rd ed. Rosemont, IL: American Academy of Orthopedic Surgeons; 2004:503-505, 541-555.

CASE 2: TRAUMATIC ABOVE KNEE AMPUTATION

A 32-year-old male with traumatic right transfemoral amputation presents 4 weeks after surgery for prosthetic prescription. His surgical site is well healed and he is ambulating with crutches indoors and outdoors for moderate distances. He has minimal residual limb or phantom limb pain.

Questions

1. What further information would you like from the patient about his previous functional activity to assist with formulating the prosthetic prescription?

2. On examination, he has a long residual limb with a well-healed surgical site. He has a tapered shape and is non-tender to palpation. What level of strength and range of motion at the right hip are necessary to resume independent ambulation in the community without an assistive device?

3. The most critical feature of prosthetic fitting is socket design and comfort. This patient had a fairly sedentary work activity level, but enjoyed recreational sports regularly including golf, basketball, and swimming. As you write the prosthetic prescription, what type of socket design and suspension would you consider for a high activity level, younger amputee?

4. Prosthetic component selection is directed by the patient's functional level and expected activities. What category of prosthetic knee and foot would be most appropriate?

5. Certain higher-level activities require special adaptations or special prosthetic devices. How will this patient resume driving and swimming?

6. Describe to the patient in lay terms how a hydraulic knee works.

7. As this same patient ages over many years, his functional status will also change. At what age should his prosthetic componentry be downgraded?

CASE 2: TRAUMATIC ABOVE KNEE AMPUTATION

Answers

1. Work activities: How far does he need to walk? Are there stairs or uneven terrain? Does he do any lifting or carrying? Does he need to drive?
Home activities: Home set-up, stairs, family responsibilities/children?
Social/recreational activities: Sports, fitness, exercise

2. Grade 4/5 strength at right hip extension and abduction is necessary to maintain trunk stability in single limb stance during ambulation (without an assistive device). Hip extension to 20° to 30° is necessary to achieve reciprocal gait with near normal gait parameters.

3. Contemporary sockets for transfemoral amputation should include a narrow mediolateral, ischial containment socket using a rigid outer frame and flexible inner socket. True suction suspension with no soft interface (skin against inner plastic socket) may give the most intimate fit and best feedback to the patient, but is very dependent on stable residual limb volume. Suction suspension using a gel liner with a strap, pin, or seal will also provide excellent suspension, and is less dependent on a stable limb volume. Semi-suction with socks and a belt provides the least effective suspension.

4. To achieve variable cadence (slow and fast walk, run), swing and stance phase control, and good stability on uneven terrain, this patient should have a hydraulic knee or microprocessor hydraulic knee. He will require a dynamic response foot (carbon fiber) to provide effective propulsion during fast walk and higher-level activities. He may also need a shock/torque absorber for high level activities with impact.

5. Return to driving after right lower limb loss requires installation of a left side gas pedal in the car and proper driver training to resume safe and legal driving. Return to swimming in a pool is best accomplished with no prosthesis in the water. Even a waterproof prosthesis does not improve swimming in a pool. However, wading into the ocean or a lake requires 2 feet on the ground; therefore, a waterproof prosthesis would be necessary in these cases.

6. A hydraulic knee has a piston, containing fluid, which controls the motion of the knee. This piston allows for variable speeds of gait, making it useful for uneven surfaces or quick changes in position.

7. Age should have little or no impact on the decision-making process for prosthetic componentry. If the patient continues to prove to be a successful prosthetic user for higher-level activities, then you should continue to prescribe the appropriate devices. The components should match the activity, not the age.

BIBLIOGRAPHY

Edelstein JE, Moroz A. *Lower-Limb Prosthetics and Orthotics: Clinical Concepts.* Thorofare, NJ: SLACK; 2011.
Esquenazi A. Amputation rehabilitation and prosthetic restoration. From surgery to community reintegration. *Disabil Rehabil.* 2004;26:831-836.
Smith DG, Michael JW, Bowker JH. *Atlas of Amputations and Limb Deficiencies: Surgical, Prosthetic, and Rehabilitation Principles.* 3rd ed. Rosemont, IL: American Academy of Orthopedic Surgeons; 2004:503-505, 541-555.

CASE 3: UPPER LIMB AMPUTATION

A 34-year-old carpenter severed his right forearm below the elbow in a work injury 3 weeks ago. He is referred to your prosthetic clinic by his trauma surgeon.

Questions

1. What further questions do you have about his history that would help you prescribe a prosthesis for him? What are important key elements in the physical exam?

2. The limb was severed by a motorized saw. His pain is reasonably well controlled with oxycodone and naproxen. He has phantom sensations but no phantom pain. He is right hand dominant. He has no significant past medical history. He wants to eventually return to work as a carpenter. He enjoys hunting, fishing, and canoeing. Workers compensation is paying for his medical care and rehabilitation after this injury. His incision is well healed and sutures have been removed. The amputation is at 5 cm from the olecranon process. There is no point tenderness. Elbow flexion and extension strength are 4/5. He has approximately 45° of pronation and supination. What diagnostic tests are indicated at this time?

3. What are the major considerations in prescribing a prosthesis for this man?

4. What are the key components of a below elbow (transradial) prosthesis? What special adaptations would help make the prosthesis more functional for him?

5. His workers compensation insurance case manager comes to the appointment with the patient. She requests to be present in the exam room during your evaluation. How should you handle this?

6. How does workers compensation insurance coverage differ from medical insurance coverage in terms of the prosthesis?

CASE 3: UPPER LIMB AMPUTATION

Answers

1. What are his vocational and recreational goals? How is his pain, and does he have phantom pain? Hand dominance? Comorbidities? On physical exam, how is the incision healing? What is the length of the residual limb? How is his elbow range and strength?

2. No diagnostic tests are necessary now. If he had point tenderness or palpable masses in the residual limb, a forearm x-ray to look for bony fragments or foreign objects could be considered.

3. He wishes to return to manual labor and outdoor sportsmen activities. A manually powered prosthesis may be more durable and reliable for these conditions. His residual limb is short, and that will require some adaptation to the suspension (likely a harness). Because he has limited supination and pronation, his prosthetic wrist will require these elements.

4. The prosthetic hand can be myo-electrically or body powered. The latter may be more practical for him if he intends to use it in wet conditions or for heavier activities. Body-powered terminal devices can be voluntary opening or voluntary closing devices. Voluntary opening devices are easier to use, particularly for prolonged grasp, but voluntary closing devices can apply more force or be used for finer movements. The prosthetic wrist can have friction activated supination and pronation, which rotate to supination during heavier lifting. Because his limb is short, he will likely need a harness suspension, as self-suspension with a supracondylar sleeve may not hold his prosthesis in place adequately (Figures 1.1, 1.2).

5. The patient should be asked if he is comfortable with this and informed he has the right to refuse. In most states, the workers compensation insurance does, however, have the right to review the medical records if they are paying the bills.

6. Workers compensation is required to provide any care or equipment needed for return to work. Medical insurance only needs to cover what is termed "medically necessary." Many insurance companies interpret this as the most basic prosthesis to return the patient to basic self-care functioning.

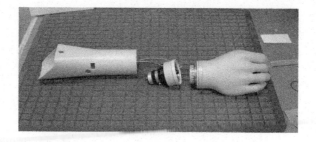

Figure 1.1 Myo-electric below-elbow prosthesis.

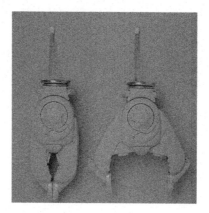

Figure 1.2 Terminal hand device that can be set as either voluntary opening (left) or voluntary closing (right).

BIBLIOGRAPHY

Edelstein JE, Moroz A. *Lower-Limb Prosthetics and Orthotics: Clinical Concepts.* Thorofare, NJ: SLACK; 2011.

Esquenazi A. Amputation rehabilitation and prosthetic restoration. From surgery to community reintegration. *Disabil Rehabil.* 2004;26:831-836.

Smith DG, Michael JW, Bowker JH. *Atlas of Amputations and Limb Deficiencies: Surgical, Prosthetic, and Rehabilitation Principles.* 3rd ed. Rosemont, IL: American Academy of Orthopedic Surgeons; 2004:503-505, 541-555.

Uustal H, Meier RH 3rd. Pain issues and treatment of the person with an amputation. *Phys Med Rehabil Clin N Am.* February 2014;25(1):45-52.

2 Brain Impairments and Central Nervous System Disorders

Michael H. Marino, Miriam Segal, and Thomas Watanabe

CASE 1: HYPOXIC BRAIN INJURY

A 22-year-old female suffered respiratory and circulatory arrest secondary to status asthmaticus. She was resuscitated by emergency medical service and subsequently hospitalized for 4 weeks with multiple complications including ventilator-dependent respiratory failure requiring tracheostomy and gastrostomy tube placement. After being weaned from the ventilator it is apparent that she has severe neurologic impairment. You are asked to see her to determine if she is a candidate for inpatient brain injury rehabilitation.

Questions

1. What are the key elements of the history?

2. The patient is awake and breathing spontaneously on humidified oxygen via tracheostomy collar. Vital signs are normal. What are the important features of the physical exam?

3. She is able to track the examiner and follow some simple commands but her responses are slow. She is not vocalizing due to the tracheostomy tube but is able to mouth some words. What are your recommendations at this point?

4. In patients with severely impaired consciousness after cardiopulmonary resuscitation, what are the key negative prognostic indicators?

5. Several months later, you see the patient for an outpatient visit. She was discharged from inpatient rehabilitation and then completed a course of outpatient physical therapy, occupational therapy, and speech therapy. She is able to walk without assistance and is performing basic activities of daily living on her own, but her family is still providing 24-hour supervision and they manage her appointments and finances. They note that sometimes they still need to cue her for safety or to complete a task. She would like to go back to school and resume driving. What are your recommendations at this point?

6. The parents are seeking legal guardianship for the patient. They bring in a form from their attorney, which asks whether the patient has capacity. How might you determine this?

CASE 1: HYPOXIC BRAIN INJURY

Answers

1. In patients with hypoxic brain injury (HBI), a complete history includes a detailed hospital course, injury mechanism, duration of hypoxia/ischemia, duration of disordered consciousness and posthypoxic amnesia, residual impairments, and medical comorbidities thus far. In terms of pre-morbid history, it is important to obtain prior functional status (including vocational history and driving), level of education, previous history of drug or alcohol abuse, previous psychiatric history and premorbid personality, as well as social support.

2. Arousal, visual tracking, response to tactile or painful stimulation, ability to follow verbal commands, ability to accurately indicate yes/no responses, passive and active range of motion in the limbs to evaluate for spasticity, contracture, or heterotopic ossification. In patients who can participate further the following should also be assessed: cerebellar and fine motor testing, coordination, visual testing (including testing for agnosia), orientation, attention, processing speed, memory, judgment, insight, affect, and behavior.

3. Initiate a multidisciplinary rehabilitation program to promote physical and cognitive recovery. This should include attention to sleep-wake cycle, management of any agitation, tracheostomy tube weaning, management of any posthypoxic seizures or movement disorders, spasticity management and serial examinations to exclude new pathology, or improvement to guide the rehabilitation program. Rehabilitation nursing involvement is important to care for skin and for bowel and bladder management as well as to help maintain the therapeutic milieu and advance team goals. Physical therapy is important for functional mobility and may address spasticity or dyskinesias as well. Occupational therapy may introduce adaptive strategies for visual and cognitive deficits as well as self-care skills. Speech/language pathology will need to work on diet advancement as well as cognitive-linguistic deficits. A neuropsychologist can help to guide the team's efforts and provide counseling and education to the patient and family. Social work is important to coordinate transitions of care, identify resources, and keep families informed of the expected course as the patient progresses through the rehabilitation process.

4. In patients with absent pupillary or corneal reflexes, or absent extensor motor responses 3 days after cardiac arrest, the outcome is invariably poor (Level A, strong evidence). A poor prognosis is also conferred if there is myoclonic status epilepticus within the first day (Level B, good evidence), bilaterally absent N20 response by day 3, or serum neuron-specific enolase (NSE) levels >33 mcg/L at days 1 to 3 (Level B, good evidence). Prognosis cannot be based on circumstances of cardiopulmonary resuscitation, elevated temperature, EEG, intracranial pressure, or neuroimaging studies.

5. Management of chronic hypoxic brain injury involves gradual reintegration into the community with ongoing education and support as well as appropriate

referrals to community-based services. This may include neuropsychological evaluation and counseling or follow up, vocational rehabilitation services, and driving evaluation if the patient is able. It is important to note that any post-hypoxic seizures may affect restoration of driving privileges. You should continue to follow up to monitor for secondary conditions such as depression or other mood disturbances.

6. Capacity means that the patient has adequate intellectual abilities to describe his or her medical situation, appraise alternatives, and make rational choices based on values. You might ask the patient to describe his or her diagnosis and treatment. You might ask what would happen if the patient did not take prescribed medications or follow through with therapies. A patient does not need to have normal intellectual function in order to have capacity.

BIBLIOGRAPHY

Eslinger PJ, Zapela G, Chakara F, Barrett AM. Cognitive impairments. In: Zasler ND, et al., eds. *Brain Injury Medicine*. 2nd ed. New York, NY: Demos Medical; 2013:chap 51.

Kothari S, DiTommaso C. Prognosis after severe traumatic brain injury: a practical, evidence-based approach. In: Zasler ND, et al., eds. *Brain Injury Medicine*. 2nd ed. New York, NY: Demos Medical; 2013.

Wang E, Schultz B. Hypoxic brain injury. *PM&R Knowledge Now*. 2012. Available at: http://me.aapmr.org/kn/article.html?id=15.

Wijdicks EFM, Hijra A, Young GB, et al. Practice parameter: prediction of outcome in comatose survivors after cardiopulmonary resuscitation (an evidence-based review). Report of the Quality Standards Subcommittee of the American Academy of Neurology. *Neurology*. 2006;6:203-210.

CASE 2: SEVERE TRAUMATIC BRAIN INJURY

A 21-year-old male is being admitted to acute rehabilitation after being treated in acute care for a traumatic brain injury and several rib fractures due to a motor vehicle crash. The patient does not have any past medical history.

Questions

1. What key elements would you want to know from the history of this injury? What information would you like to have from pre-injury history?

2. The records indicate that the injury occurred in a high-speed motor vehicle crash and that your patient was the driver. His initial Glasgow Coma Scale score was 6 and his trauma workup revealed bifrontal contusions and diffuse subarachnoid hemorrhage as well as multiple rib fractures. He was intubated and sedated and had an intracranial pressure monitor placed. One week later he was extubated and transferred to a step-down floor where he had some intermittent fevers and tachycardia without an infectious source. It is now 3 weeks postinjury and he remains nonverbal. What is important to look for on physical exam?

3. The patient is awake and appears alert. He visually tracks the examiner and pushes the examiner away with painful stimulation. His psychomotor activity is slightly increased. He does not follow any verbal commands or indicate a yes/no response. What is the level of severity of this patient's traumatic brain injury? What are some important prognostic indicators in a patient such as this? What assessment instruments would be helpful in forecasting this patient's recovery?

4. The patient transitions to your acute rehabilitation unit. What pharmacologic interventions would you consider to improve recovery?

5. Over the next few months the patient completes inpatient and out-patient rehabilitation. He recovers basic language skills and is able to ambulate; however, he has significant residual cognitive deficits and requires partial supervision from family. He is interested in returning to work and driving. How can you help him? What are some good predictors of success?

6. The patient does poorly with his driver evaluation, and is distraught over the results. How can you counsel him regarding avoidance of driving?

CASE 2: SEVERE TRAUMATIC BRAIN INJURY

Answers

1. Certain elements of the injury's history will help to determine injury severity as well as the pattern of deficits that would be expected and the prognosis for a good recovery. These would be injury mechanism, loss of consciousness and duration, residual impairments (especially posttraumatic amnesia), initial Glasgow Coma Scale score, associated injuries, and postinjury complications thus far. Certain elements of the pre-injury history are useful in the course of recovery. These would be prior functional status (including vocational history and driving), level of education, previous history of drug or alcohol abuse, previous psychiatric history, previous history of traumatic brain injury, social supports, and premorbid personality.

2. Important elements of a physical exam in such a case are: arousal, visual tracking, response to tactile or painful stimulation, ability to follow verbal commands, ability to accurately indicate yes/no responses, orientation if possible, passive and active range of motion in the limbs as best as can possibly be assessed if the patient cannot follow commands, as well as tone.

3. This patient has a severe traumatic brain injury. Since his level of consciousness seems to be impaired, the Coma Recovery Scale-Revised (CRS-R) can be used to predict recovery. As he emerges, the Galveston Orientation and Amnesia Test (GOAT) or the Orientation-log (O-log) can be used to assess posttraumatic amnesia (PTA). A patient is considered emerged from PTA with a score >75 on the GOAT or >25 on the O-log for 2 consecutive days. Early predictors of recovery are time to follow commands (also defined as length of coma), duration of PTA, and age. Individuals greater than 65 years old are not likely to have a "good" recovery, meaning little to no disability.

4. Before adding any pharmacologic agents to improve recovery, the list of active medications should be reviewed and any medications that potentially impair cognition should be discontinued or weaned. This may include opiates, benzodiazepines, antipsychotics, and medications with anticholinergic activity. If the patient is on anticonvulsants, the need to continue them should be evaluated. For patients with posttraumatic disorders of consciousness, amantadine has been demonstrated to accelerate the pace of functional recovery.

5. Now that the patient has made a good physical recovery and has been discharged from outpatient therapies it is time to refer him to home- and community-based rehabilitation services that can eventually include vocational rehabilitation and an assessment by a certified driving rehabilitation specialist to determine his readiness to resume driving. Patients who have supportive families or significant others are more likely to succeed and so involving them is very important.

6. Be empathetic and acknowledge his frustration. Driving puts him at risk of injuring not only himself but others. In many states, you as a physician may be obligated to report him to the motor vehicle administration. You should engage his family for help in enforcing this restriction, as well as in counseling him about the risks.

BIBLIOGRAPHY

Kothari S, DiTommaso C. Prognosis after severe traumatic brain injury: a practical, evidence-based approach. In: Zasler ND, et al., eds. *Brain Injury Medicine*. 2nd ed. New York, NY: Demos Medical; 2013.

Malec JF. Posthospital rehabilitation. In: Zasler ND, et al., eds. *Brain Injury Medicine*. 2nd ed. New York, NY: Demos Medical; 2013.

Wolf C, McLaughlin M, Khadavi M, et al. Traumatic brain injury. *PM&R Knowledge Now*. 2015. Available at: http://me.aapmr.org/kn/article.html?id=41.

Wortzel HS, Arcineigas DB. Treatment of post-traumatic cognitive impairments. *Curr Treat Options Neurol.* 2012;14(5):493-508.

Yudolfsky SC, Silver JM, Anderson KE. Aggressive disorders. In: Arcineigas DB, et al., eds. *Management of Adults With Traumatic Brain Injury*. Arlington, VA: American Psychiatric Association; 2013:chap 10.

CASE 3: ACUTE CONCUSSION

A 17-year-old high school student is seen in the clinic 3 days after being removed from a football game by the athletic trainer due to a suspected concussion. He reports having had no prior concussions.

Questions

1. What history and physical findings are important in determining whether he has had a significant concussion?

2. You learn that he had some momentary loss of consciousness and disorientation on the field. Today he still has a headache, and reports difficulty concentrating in class. His Mini-Mental Status Exam is 28/30. He was admitted to a hospital overnight after sustaining a traumatic brain injury with 10-minute loss of consciousness from a fall when he was 10 years old. What information may lead you to conclude that this player may be at risk for a prolonged recovery time?

3. How should you proceed regarding clearance for return to play?

4. His mother asks about whether his prior traumatic brain injury puts him at increased risk for chronic traumatic encephalopathy (CTE). How do you respond?

5. The following day, the boy's football coach calls. He wants him to play in next week's homecoming game, as the patient is the star quarterback. How should you respond?

6. The patient has a major exam next week, and he is worried about his performance. What can be done to help him with this issue?

CASE 3: ACUTE CONCUSSION

Answers

1. One should determine if there was any loss of consciousness, although one can have a concussion without this. Amnesia, altered level of alertness, behavioral changes, fatigue, nausea, headache, and balance problems are all common symptoms. Ideally, the athlete should be examined immediately on the field for changes in orientation, alertness, cranial nerve findings, and balance, coordination, and motor deficits. However, high schools frequently do not have the resources to do this, so it should be done in the office when seen by the physician. A Mini-Mental Status Exam should be performed. One should ask about any prior history of head injuries.

2. Certain findings are predictive of higher risk for delayed recovery time: visual memory and processing speed problems, migraine headaches, complaints of "fogginess," and multiple prior concussions.

3. Return to play should follow a stepwise protocol. Do not initiate activity until the athlete is asymptomatic at rest. Then, increase level of intensity in non-contact activity (light exercise, moderate exercise, then heavy exercise, then contact in practice, finally full clearance for game play). If the athlete develops symptoms at any level, return to the prior asymptomatic activity level and proceed as tolerated. The athlete should have returned to the prior level of neurocognitive function prior to return to play as well.

4. The prior traumatic brain injury is only one of the multiple factors that may lead to chronic traumatic encephalopathy (CTE). CTE may be related to the cumulative number of subconcussive blows that an athlete receives, the number of concussions, genetic factors, and environmental factors.

5. Because of HIPAA laws, you cannot speak to the coach without written consent from the patient and his parent(s). If they do provide consent, you should emphasize that your professional duty is to the patient's health, and that you will not change your recommendations based on the needs of the team.

6. You can talk to the school and see if they are willing to either postpone the exam or perhaps allow the patient more time to complete the exam. Usually to qualify for accommodations under the law, a student would need to have a certified disability and an individualized education plan in place. These are not usually done for a temporary disability. However, the teacher or principal may be willing to accommodate under these circumstances.

BIBLIOGRAPHY

Aligene K, Lin E. Vestibular and balance treatment of the concussed athlete. *NeuroRehabilation*. 2013;32(3):543-553.

Collins M, Iverson GL, Gaetz MB, Meehan WP, Lowell MR. Sports related concussion. In: Zasler ND, et al., eds. *Brain Injury Medicine*. 2nd ed. New York, NY: Demos Medical; 2013:chap 31.

McCrory P, Meeuwisse WH, Aubry M, et al. Consensus agreement statement of the 4th International Conference on concussion in sport. *J Am Coll Surg*. May 2013;216(5):e55-e71.

CASE 4: POSTCONCUSSIVE SYNDROME

A 40-year-old female is referred to you by her attorney for lingering symptoms related to a motor vehicle crash 6 months prior.

Questions

1. What details of the accident are helpful in determining the severity of her injury?

2. She had no loss of consciousness and took herself to the emergency department, where she had a Glasgow Coma Scale score of 15 and an unremarkable head CT. What pre-injury risk factors may have contributed to this slow recovery despite lack of severity of findings on initial presentation?

3. She reports that she has had persistent headaches. What approach should be taken to assess and manage posttraumatic headaches?

4. Dizziness is a prominent symptom with accompanying balance problems. What are the common reasons for these symptoms after mild TBI and how do they present?

5. Discuss the role of posttraumatic psychosocial factors in delaying recovery.

6. Her attorney asks if this is a case of postconcussive syndrome. How do you respond?

CASE 4: POSTCONCUSSIVE SYNDROME

Answers

1. Important details from the acute injury are any loss of consciousness, Glasgow Coma Scale score, and radiographic results (CT scan?).

2. Personality characteristics, mental health problems, substance abuse, prior brain injuries, and prior medical/neurologic problems are all important factors in predisposing the patient to chronic postconcussive symptoms.

3. Assess prior history of headaches. Categorize the headache. Determine interventions based on headache type. Migrainous headaches are most common, followed by tension-type headaches. Occipital neuralgia is also common. Migraines are episodic, often have auras or visual changes, and are described as throbbing or pounding. Tension headaches are more constant, and frequently originate from the neck or occiput. With occipital neuralgia, there is a Tinel's sign over the greater or lesser occipital nerves, reproducing symptoms.

4. Benign paroxysmal positional vertigo is demonstrated with rapid changes in position, and, specifically, by performing the Dix-Halpike maneuver. Posttraumatic perilymphatic fistula may present with vertigo, fluctuating hearing loss, tinnitus, nausea, and postexertional headache. Posttraumatic endolymphatic hydrops is associated with ipsilateral low frequency hearing loss and a sensation of ear fullness.

5. Physical, emotional, cognitive, vocational, financial, and recreational factors may all play a role in delaying recovery. They may lead to maladaptive health-related beliefs that may be difficult to treat.

6. You should explain your findings in lay terms. To meet the criteria for postconcussive syndrome the patient must have a history of head trauma, and findings in at least three of six areas: (a) headache, dizziness, fatigue, noise intolerance; (b) emotional changes; (c) subjective cognitive complaints; (d) insomnia; (e) reduced alcohol tolerance; and (f) preoccupation with symptoms, fear of permanent brain damage, or adoption of the sick role.

BIBLIOGRAPHY

Aligene K, Lin E. Vestibular and balance treatment of the concussed athlete. *NeuroRehabilation*. 2013;32(3):543-553.
Iverson GL, Lange RT, Gaetz MB, Zasler ND. Mild traumatic brain injury. In: Zasler ND, et al., eds. *Brain Injury Medicine*. 2nd ed. New York, NY: Demos Medical; 2013:chap 29.
Wortzel HS, Arcineigas DB. Treatment of post-traumatic cognitive impairments. *Curr Treat Options Neurol.* 2012;14(5):493-508.

CASE 5: BEHAVIORAL MANAGEMENT

A 23-year-old male is admitted to the inpatient brain injury rehabilitation unit after sustaining a traumatic brain injury due to a high-speed motor vehicle crash 2 weeks ago. He is awake and alert but confused and disoriented. He is uncooperative with treatments and at times aggressive.

Questions

1. What more do you need to know about his history in regard to these behavioral problems?

2. He had no premorbid history of behavioral problems. He had bilateral frontotemporal intracerebral hemorrhages on his CT at the time of his injury. He has no relevant comorbidities. What nonpharmacologic approaches may help decrease his agitation?

3. What classes of medications could be considered to control his behavior and what side effects should be considered for each class?

4. To determine whether your interventions are effective, what validated outcome measures can be used?

5. A nursing assistant comes to you extremely angry. She says the patient became sexually aggressive with her, exposing himself and using profane language. She no longer wants to care for the patient. How can you help defuse the situation?

6. A nurse comes to you reporting the patient is punching staff members, and wants an order for hand restraints. What policies must you keep in mind before ordering restraints?

CASE 5: BEHAVIORAL MANAGEMENT

Answers

1. One would want to know if he had any premorbid behavioral issues or psychiatric disorders. The location of his brain injury is also important; agitation is most frequently associated with orbito-frontal injuries. These commonly occur in acceleration/deceleration mechanism of injury (e.g., high-speed motor vehicle crashes) due to the rough undersurface of the skull in this region. The nursing and therapy staff should be interviewed to determine triggers for the behavior, as well as its severity. Is the patient at risk for harming himself or others? One must assess for comorbidities such as infections, metabolic disorders, hypoxia, electrolyte abnormalities, sleep deficits, or seizures that may contribute.

2. Avoid overstimulation (e.g., crowded rooms, or television), provide day/night cues, orientation cues, and quiet at night. Having a family member stay with him can be helpful. If he is at risk of falling, a sitter may reduce that risk, as can video surveillance, if available. Restraints should be avoided, as these can both increase agitation and also be risk factors for more serious injury. Minimize invasive devices such as IVs or Foley catheters as much as possible.

3. Medications should be used only when conservative measures are failing and the patient is at risk of injuring himself or others. Some medications and possible side effects include antipsychotics (sedation, slowing of motor recovery, QT interval prolongation, epileptogenic), beta-blockers (hypotension, sedation), antiseizure medications (hepatotoxicity, sedation), lithium (renal problems), and serotonergic medications (electrolyte abnormalities, serotonin syndrome, and priapism).

4. Agitated Behavioral Scale (ABS), Overt Agitation Severity Scale (OASS), or Overt Behaviour Scale (OBS).

5. Staff on a brain injury unit should be trained about common behavioral problems in this population and have basic understanding of the physiology behind these issues. Sexually aggressive behavior should be treated by establishing firm limits, without escalating emotional responses. The psychologist may help develop cognitive behavioral approaches including appropriate rewards and punishments to suppress these behaviors.

6. Physical restraints should be used only as a last resort if the patient is a risk to self or others. Most regulatory bodies (Joint Commission or Commission on Accreditation of Rehabilitation Facilities) require clear hospital policies that address when restraints can be used, duration of use, frequent reassessment of the necessity of restraints (usually at least daily), and documentation of why alternatives could not be used.

BIBLIOGRAPHY

Eslinger PJ, et al. Cognitive impairments. In: Zasler ND, et al., eds. *Brain Injury Medicine*. 2nd ed. New York, NY: Demos Medical; 2013:chap 51.

Wolf C, McLaughlin M, Khadavi M, et al. Traumatic brain injury. *PM&R Knowledge Now*. 2015. Available at: http://me.aapmr.org/kn/article.html?id=41.

Wortzel HS, Arcineigas DB. Treatment of post-traumatic cognitive impairments. *Curr Treat Options Neurol*. 2012; 14(5):493-508.

Yudolfsky SC, Silver JM, Anderson KE. Aggressive disorders. In: Archinegos DB, Zasler ND, Vanderplog RD, Jaffee MS, eds. *Management of Adults With Traumatic Brain Injury*. Arlington, VA: American Psychiatric Association; 2013:chap 10.

CASE 6: OUTPATIENT MANAGEMENT

A 45-year-old college professor fell down a flight of stairs when leaving the lecture hall and sustained a traumatic brain injury. He was admitted to a hospital and was discharged after 2 days. He was referred to be seen in the PM&R clinic 2 weeks later.

Questions

1. What questions should you ask him to determine if he is having ongoing disability from this injury? What exam should be done?

2. He notes that he has difficulty concentrating and staying on task, and is easily distracted. He denies vertigo, balance or coordination problems, and has no headache or visual symptoms. His Mini-Mental Status Exam score is 28/30. What concurrent problems associated with his brain injury may be leading to or exacerbating these complaints?

3. Explain the effects of concussion to him.

4. He has heard that comprehensive neuropsychological testing is the definitive way to diagnose cognitive deficits and asks whether you will order this soon. How do you respond to this assertion and the question regarding timing?

5. He has taken the remainder of the semester off work. Two months after his injury, he is continuing to demonstrate deficits in arousal, attention, and processing speed. What class of medications may be most appropriate to help address this problem, and what are their potential side effects?

6. How could you determine his readiness to return to work? What resources might be available to assist in this process?

CASE 6: OUTPATIENT MANAGEMENT

Answers

1. One should ask about difficulties with memory, attention, emotional lability, mood, headaches, vision, balance, and coordination. The Mini-Mental Status Examination (MMSE) and Montreal Cognitive Assessment (MoCA) are simple cognitive screening tools. A standard neurologic exam including cranial nerves, finger-nose-finger, and gait evaluation should be performed.

2. Poor sleep, medications, headaches, visual problems, anxiety, and depression can contribute to cognitive dysfunction.

3. Because he is a professor, your language can be at a higher level, but you still need to avoid medical jargon. Concussion is a "bruising" of the brain. You do not necessarily need loss of consciousness to have a concussion. Effects may last from a few days to permanent damage depending on the severity. Patients often have headaches, visual problems, cognitive difficulties, mood disturbance, insomnia, or excessive sleepiness.

4. Neuropsychological testing is the most sensitive measure of cognitive function. That is not to say that it can definitively diagnose a concussion, although patterns of deficits identified may help suggest consistency with traumatic brain injury. If it is important early on to determine whether the patient has subtle deficits that might be clinically important and not easily detectable by other means, early neuropsychological testing may be indicated. It should also be noted that some elements of neuropsychological tests may not be able to be repeated for several months, so if a re-evaluation is needed, it may need to be delayed.

5. The class of medications that may be most beneficial are stimulant medications. Potential side effects include anxiety/nervousness, decreased appetite, and elevations in heart rate and blood pressure.

6. One needs to know the details of his job duties. Is he giving lectures, teaching small groups, doing research, writing, or doing administrative work? In addition to cognitive testing, more functionally based tests may be useful to evaluate specific work-related tasks. These may be performed by occupational therapy or a speech language pathologist. If the injury is work-related, benefits will also be available through workers compensation. A case manager may be able to get him vocational counseling and also work with his employer on reasonable accommodations.

BIBLIOGRAPHY

Aligene K, Lin E. Vestibular and balance treatment of the concussed athlete. *NeuroRehabilitation.* 2013;32(3):543-553.
Iverson GL, et al. Mild traumatic brain injury. In: Zasler ND, et al., eds. *Brain Injury Medicine.* 2nd ed. New York, NY: Demos Medical; 2013:chap 29.
Wortzel HS, Arcineigas DB. Treatment of post-traumatic cognitive impairments. *Curr Treat Options Neurol.* 2012;14(5):493-508.

CASE 7: COMPLICATIONS OF TRAUMATIC BRAIN INJURY

A 48-year-old man who suffered a gunshot wound to the head is in your acute inpatient rehabilitation unit. He had a right-sided decompressive craniectomy 8 weeks ago and has left hemiparesis. A nurse informs you he is more lethargic than usual this morning with difficulty waking up. At baseline he is alert, responsive, and appropriate.

Questions

1. What specific information do you want to know about his course overnight?

2. You learn that he slept well, no medication changes were made, and he was afebrile with stable vitals. You go to examine the patient. What is critical to do on physical exam?

3. You find that he is answering questions but is lethargic and slow to respond. His craniectomy site appears slightly more tense and bulging than you remembered. What is your differential diagnosis?

4. What workup would you order?

5. His seizure, metabolic, and infectious workup is negative. CT of the head shows a hydrocephalus and he is sent for shunt placement. What are the types of hydrocephalus and which is more common in traumatic brain injury? What are possible complications that can arise related to a ventriculoperitoneal (VP) shunt?

6. Explain to his wife what hydrocephalus is in lay terms.

7. How might you go about establishing guidelines on your brain injury unit for monitoring patients for hydrocephalus?

CASE 7: COMPLICATIONS OF TRAUMATIC BRAIN INJURY

Answers

1. You should ask about any recent medication changes or missed doses. His sleep-wake cycle should be explored. Has he had any symptoms of infection such as cough or dysuria?

2. Begin with checking vital signs and his level of arousal/responsiveness. Examine the craniectomy site for subgaleal effusion or incisional erythema. Test pupillary reactions and eye movements, strength, sensation, and muscle tone. Observe for signs of shaking/seizures.

3. Differential diagnosis includes metabolic/electrolyte disturbance, rebleeding/ intracranial hemorrhage, hydrocephalus, seizure, central nervous system infection (abscess or meningitis), and urinary tract infection.

4. Labs and tests would include basic metabolic panel (BMP), CBC with differential, urinalysis, CT head, and EEG.

5. Types of hydrocephalus are communicating versus noncommunicating (obstructive) hydrocephalus. Communicating hydrocephalus is more common. Potential complications of VP shunts are infection, undershunting (or shunt failure), overshunting (which can cause intracranial hemorrhage), headache, and seizures.

6. You should explain in lay terms that hydrocephalus (Figure 2.1) is excess fluid in the brain, caused by obstruction of flow. The effects of hydrocephalus on cognition, gait, and continence should be explained.

7. Do a plan, do, see, act (PDSA) cycle. Perform a literature review for identifying subpopulations at risk for developing hydrocephalus (plan). Educate staff about signs and symptoms of hydrocephalus (do). See how many hydrocephalus cases are identified in your unit over a quarter, and whether they were found early (see). Then determine if further interventions, such as order sets, are needed (act).

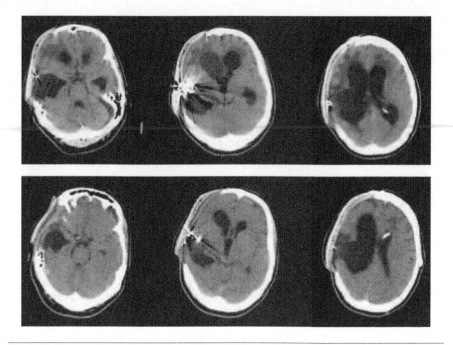

Figure 2.1 Hydrocephalus.
Source: From Zasler ND, et al., eds. *Brain Injury Medicine.* 2nd ed. New York, NY: Demos Medical; 2013.

BIBLIOGRAPHY

Long DF. Diagnosis and management of late intracranial complications of TBI. In: Zasler ND, et al., eds. *Brain Injury Medicine.* 2nd ed. New York, NY: Demos Medical; 2013:chap 44.
Wolf C, McLaughlin M, Khadavi M, et al. Traumatic brain injury. *PM&R Knowledge Now.* 2015. Available at: http://me.aapmr.org/kn/article.html?id=41.

CASE 8: PARKINSON'S DISEASE

A 65-year-old woman is seen in your clinic. She has a family history of idiopathic Parkinson's disease and she is concerned that she is developing symptoms.

Questions

1. What elements of history and physical exam are critical in making a diagnosis of Parkinson's disease?

2. What is the differential diagnosis for Parkinson's disease?

3. Your patient has early signs of Parkinson's disease on exam and may be a candidate for pharmacologic therapy. Are there any medications that can alter the course of the disease?

4. Parkinson's disease is a progressive neurodegenerative disease. What is the role of rehabilitation?

5. What are the surgical treatments for advanced Parkinson's disease?

6. Her mother died after a prolonged course of Parkinson's disease. She would like to be assured that if/when her mental condition deteriorates, she does not go through what her mother did. What advice do you have?

7. What home modifications should she consider?

CASE 8: PARKINSON'S DISEASE

Answers

1. Signs and symptoms include resting tremor, bradykinesia, rigidity, masked facies, festinating gait, postural instability, freezing episodes, cognitive changes, orthostasis, micrographia, and low voice volume.

2. Exposure to medications including neuroleptics, metoclopramide, lithium, and amiodarone can cause these symptoms. Complications of traumatic brain injuries, stroke, brain tumor, and metabolic encephalopathy can also mimic Parkinson's disease.

3. There is no conclusive evidence to support the use of any medications to significantly alter the course of the disease. However, symptoms can be controlled with dopaminergic agents. Levodopa/carbidopa is a combination medication commonly prescribed for Parkinson's disease. Levodopa raises dopamine levels by serving as the metabolic precursor to dopamine. Carbidopa prevents systemic metabolism of levodopa.

4. Rehabilitation can be effective in the short term in improving gait, activities of daily living, speech quality, cognition, providing adaptive equipment, and improving home safety. Gains made in rehabilitation are lost over time so patients should be sent to physical, occupational, and speech therapy every 6 to 12 months.

5. There are two broad categories of neurosurgical procedures used currently. Destructive surgery includes thalamotomy or pallidotomy. Deep brain stimulation using electrodes implanted in the substantia nigra can help with tremor.

6. She should write a living will or prepare advance directives. She should identify a person to be her durable power of attorney should she become mentally incapacitated, and make sure that person knows her wishes not only about resuscitation, but also mechanical ventilation, enteral nutrition, life-prolonging medications, dialysis, and rehospitalizations.

7. If possible, she should live in a one-story home. She should minimize obstructions. Area rugs should be taped down. Her bathroom should have grab bars or a 3-in-1 commode. She should have night lights.

BIBLIOGRAPHY

Ropper AH, Samuels MA, Klein JP, ed. *Degenerative Diseases of the Nervous System. Adams and Victor's Principles of Neurology.* 10th ed. China: McGraw-Hill; 2014:chap 39.

Saulino M, Doherty J, Fried G. Rehabilitation concerns in degenerative movement disorders of the central nervous system. In: Braddom RL, ed. *Physical Medicine and Rehabilitation.* 3rd ed. Philadelphia, PA: Saunders; 2007:chap 52.

Vercueil L. Fifty years of brain surgery for dystonia: Revisiting the Irving S. Cooper's legacy, and looking forward. *Acta Neurol Belg.* 2003;103:125-128.

CASE 9: MULTIPLE SCLEROSIS

A 27-year-old woman has had multiple sclerosis (MS) for 5 years. She is finding it more difficult to walk recently over the summer. She is on a beta-interferon but takes no other medications. Her last acute flare was 2 years ago. Vitals are normal.

Questions

1. What key elements do you want to know from her history? What complications of MS do you need to ask about in your review of systems?

2. She tells you that this has been a gradual insidious worsening, mainly due to stiffness in her legs. She also fatigues easily. She has had some urinary incontinence recently. What is critical to do on physical exam?

3. Mental status, cranial nerves, sensation, and coordination are intact. Strength is 5/5, but she has modified Ashworth scale 2 tone in her lower limbs, especially adductors, ankle plantar flexion, and inversion. She has three beats of clonus in both ankles. Her gait is a spastic diplegic pattern. Range of motion at hips, knees, and ankles is full. Skin is intact. What is the differential diagnosis of her difficulty walking? What diagnostic testing, if any, is indicated?

4. MRI shows plaques in the thoracic cord and periventricular white matter, which are unchanged from 2 years ago. Urinalysis is normal. What interventions would help her gait?

5. She works as an elementary school teacher, but is finding it difficult to continue working. She wants to apply for Social Security. What advice would you give her regarding applying for this?

6. You recommend an ankle foot orthosis, but the patient is reluctant to use this because of cosmesis. How would you try to convince her to use this device?

CASE 9: MULTIPLE SCLEROSIS

Answers

1. The course of her MS is critical to assess (relapse or insidious progression?). Review of symptoms should include: vision changes, tremor, fatigue, heat sensitivity, weakness in limbs, spasms, and bladder changes.

2. Physical exam includes cranial nerves, sensation, coordination, strength, muscle tone, reflexes, range of motion, and gait analysis.

3. Differential diagnosis: flare, secondary progressive disease, "pseudo-flare" from infection or other stressor, heat sensitivity, ataxia, spasticity. Tests: MRI, urinalysis.

4. Treatment includes physical therapy for gait training and stretching, maintaining cool environment, orthotics prescription, spasticity management, and dalfampridine (Ampyra). Corticosteroids or ACTH and plasmapheresis are not indicated as this is secondary progressive MS and not a flare.

5. Social Security requires documentation of total and permanent disability (inability to perform any kind of work for which she's educationally qualified). Discuss reasonable accommodation under the Americans with Disability Act (e.g., air conditioning, teaching while seated, teacher's aide, first floor classroom).

6. Be empathetic and acknowledge her concerns. You can discuss how an AFO can give one a more normal gait pattern, decrease risk of falling, and decrease energy of gait. You should also discuss how a molded AFO can be hidden by slacks.

BIBLIOGRAPHY

Samkoff LM, Goodman AD. Symptomatic management in multiple sclerosis. *Neurol Clin.* 2011;29(2):449-463.

Shah A, Flores A, Nourbaksh B, Stieve O. Multiple sclerosis. In: Cifu DX, ed. *Braddom's Physical Medicine and Rehabilitation.* 5th ed. Philadelphia, PA: Elsevier; 2015:1029-1052.

Cancer and Other Medically Related Impairments

Julie K. Silver and R. Samuel Mayer

CASE 1: HEAD AND NECK CANCER

A 70-year-old man presents to your cancer rehabilitation program with recently diagnosed laryngeal cancer. He is starting chemotherapy and radiation therapy, and will undergo laryngectomy and radical neck dissection in 3 weeks.

Questions

1. What additional history would you like to know? What should you focus on with your physical exam?

2. He has some hoarseness but is otherwise asymptomatic. He has mild chronic obstructive pulmonary disease, and uses an inhaler infrequently. He quit smoking 2 years ago. What should the focus of his rehabilitation be at this time?

3. He returns to your clinic postoperatively. He has had a right radical neck dissection and laryngectomy. He is aphonic. He reports neck and right shoulder pain. What is the differential diagnosis for these complaints, and what physical exam findings and diagnostic tests would help establish a diagnosis?

4. He has right inferolateral scapular winging with shoulder shrug. EMG shows positive sharp waves and large amplitude MUPs with decreased recruitment in the trapezius. What is the diagnosis and how would you treat this condition?

5. He undergoes video-fluoroscopy swallow evaluation, which demonstrates aspiration of all consistencies of liquids and solids. The speech therapist recommends that he be NPO, and should have a percutaneous endoscopically placed gastrostomy (PEG) tube. He refuses, saying food is his only joy. How should you respond?

6. You are interested in seeing more patients like this and expanding your head and neck cancer rehabilitation program. How would you go about this?

CASE 1: HEAD AND NECK CANCER

Answers

1. You would want to know his goals. He wants to enjoy his retirement, especially holidays with his grandchildren. What are his current symptoms? You ask about comorbidities. You ask if he has any side effects from his chemotherapy, especially numbness. You would want to examine his neck for lymphadenopathy and range of motion. A careful neurologic exam should include a thorough examination for cranial nerve and sensory deficits.

2. At this phase of his disease, he should engage in a "prehabilitation" program focusing on prevention of common complications. This would include swallowing exercises, strengthening, and promoting range of motion of the neck.

3. The differential diagnosis includes fibrosis of neck muscles from surgical scarring or radiation fibrosis, spinal accessory palsy, lymphedema, or brachial plexopathy. Physical exam should include range of motion, palpation for lymphedema, and observation of scapular motion during shoulder flexion and shrugging. Electrodiagnostic testing will be useful.

4. The likely diagnosis is spinal accessory nerve palsy. Physical therapy, including taping, and neuromuscular stimulation may help. Gabapentin, pregabalin, and/or a serotonin-norepinephrine reuptake inhibitor may help with neuropathic pain.

5. One should be empathetic and listen to his concerns. He is an adult and has every right to refuse the procedure. After listening, remind him that his 5-year survival with laryngeal cancer is over 50%, and that nutrition is critical to his quality of life. The enteral feedings may well be temporary until he regains strength in his pharyngeal muscles. Express your concern regarding his ability to maintain his nutrition without getting pneumonia. He can then make an informed decision.

6. Marketing the program should be targeted at the treating physicians: the otolaryngologists and medical and radiation oncologists. In addition, nurse navigators, nurse practitioners, and/or physician assistants often are the primary referring providers for these services. Attending tumor boards or cancer committee meetings help reinforce these connections.

BIBLIOGRAPHY

Aghalar MR, Custodio CM. Chemotherapy-induced peripheral neuropathy. In: Frontera WR, Silver JK, eds. *Essentials of Physical Medicine and Rehabilitation*. Philadelphia, PA: Elsevier; 2015:chap 96:482-484.

CASE 2: BREAST CANCER

A 60-year-old woman sees you for the first time and reports that 1 year ago she was diagnosed with breast cancer and underwent a right mastectomy with a sentinel lymph node biopsy followed by chemotherapy and radiation therapy. She reports that the reason she came to see you is that her right arm started swelling a week or so ago.

Questions

1. What are the most important questions in the history to help sort out the etiology?

2. Based on her history, you suspect lymphedema. Her physical examination reveals mild swelling of the right arm and hand. The extremity is soft to the touch and has pitting edema that is reversible. What diagnostic tests are helpful in ruling out causes other than lymphedema for the arm swelling?

3. What treatment regimen would you prescribe for her?

4. You diagnosed her with lymphedema 3 months ago and sent her to physical therapy. She has completed physical therapy and wants advice about going to the gym. What do you tell her about doing resistance exercises since she has lymphedema?

5. She returns 2 years later with recurrence of her lymphedema. You note that she is not wearing her compression garments. How would you approach this with her?

6. Her sleeve has worn out, and she says that she cannot afford a replacement garment, as her medical insurance will not cover this. What approaches can you offer?

CASE 2: BREAST CANCER

Answers

1. Is it painful? The hallmark of lymphedema is painless swelling, so if she says it hurts, then lymphedema is much less likely than other conditions. You should also ask about erythema, warmth, or drainage (for cellulitis). History of lymph node dissection or sentinel node biopsy makes lymphedema more likely. Late stage cancer would trigger more thought about metastasis. History of coagulopathy or atrial fibrillation might trigger thought for deep venous thrombosis.

2. A Doppler ultrasound to rule out deep venous thrombosis is warranted given the acute onset of swelling. If her breast cancer was in a more advanced stage, an MRI of the limb might help exclude metastasis.

3. Treatment includes decompressive manual therapy followed by application of compression tapes, and then prescription compression garments.

4. Resistance exercise is likely to be safe in people diagnosed with lymphedema but should be appropriately recommended. The patient should be advised how to begin and advance her program.

5. Do not assume that her noncompliance is from a lack of motivation. Her compression garments may have worn out and she may not have insurance coverage or funding to replace them. Perhaps she finds it difficult to wear them in hot weather. Ask the reasons and problem solve with her how to overcome them.

6. Compression garments are frequently not covered by insurance. Sometimes funding can be found through charitable organizations. Sometimes, you have to compromise and go with a less expensive alternative like Ace wrapping.

BIBLIOGRAPHY

Caban M, Hall L. Lymphedema. In: Frontera WR, Silver JK, Rizzo TD Jr, eds. *Essentials of Physical Medicine and Rehabilitation*. Philadelphia, PA: Elsevier; 2015: chap 131:677.

Nelson NL. Breast cancer-related lymphedema and resistance exercise: a systematic review. *J Strength Cond Res.* 2016 Sep;30(9):2656-65.

CASE 3: LEUKEMIA/CANCER-RELATED FATIGUE

A 26-year-old man was diagnosed with leukemia. He comes to see you for fatigue and problems functioning in general.

Questions

1. What questions do you want to ask him about his cancer or his oncological treatment?

2. You learn that he finished all of his treatment 6 months ago and has no known active cancer in his body. He hopes that he is cured. On review of systems, you have an opportunity to find out more about his sleep. He tells you that sleep does not help him. What is the differential diagnosis of his fatigue?

3. On physical examination, patients with cancer-related fatigue usually do not have distinctive findings. However, if your physical examination revealed proximal weakness in the upper and lower extremities, what diagnosis would you be considering?

4. Diagnostic testing for cancer-related fatigue is usually done to rule out other diagnoses. What are important systemic diagnoses to exclude?

5. Explain cancer-related fatigue to the patient in lay terms.

6. You tell the patient that he has cancer-related fatigue and that studies show one of the best treatments for this is exercise on a regular basis. He has been sedentary and wants to begin to exercise. How would you counsel him regarding the type of exercise that has been shown to work in cancer-related fatigue?

7. He has missed substantial time from his work as a plumber. He is worried about losing his job. What legal protections does he have?

CASE 3: LEUKEMIA/CANCER-RELATED FATIGUE

Answers

1. It is important to know if he is receiving active treatment and what kind. It is also important to know if he has residual cancer and whether he is deemed curable.

2. Fatigue may be from medications, anemia, chronic infection, or cardiopulmonary or neuromuscular impairments. Cancer-related fatigue is by definition a distressing and subjective sense of physical, emotional, and/or cognitive tiredness that is related to cancer or its treatment. Cancer-related fatigue is not proportional to one's activity level and often isn't responsive to rest or sleep.

3. Proximal weakness is often associated with steroid myopathy. Cancer patients are frequently treated with steroids, and if you find proximal weakness, this should be investigated further.

4. Differential diagnosis can also include depression, thyroid disease, malnutrition, anemia, insomnia, and indolent infections.

5. Cancer-related fatigue is a very common phenomenon impacting almost three fourths of cancer patients. While it can be related to chemotherapy or radiation, it often persists long after treatment is completed. Patients feel tired despite getting adequate rest. There can be difficulty concentrating. Counterintuitively, the treatment is not rest, but rather graded exercise.

6. Both cardiovascular and strength training exercise have been shown to reduce symptoms of cancer-related fatigue. Usually modest exercise intensity levels (up to 60% of maximum oxygen consumption) for 5 days per week is tolerated by patients even if they are undergoing active cancer treatment. However, appropriate precautions and contraindications should always be adhered to with all patients, particularly those in active treatment.

7. The Family Medical Leave Act provides for up to 12 weeks per year of unpaid leave from work, prohibiting employers from terminating employees if they have a documented medical condition. Once he is ready to return to work, the Americans with Disabilities Act requires employers to make reasonable accommodations as long as the employee can perform the essential job requirements.

BIBLIOGRAPHY

Cheville A. Cancer-related fatigue. In: Frontera WL, Silver JK, Rizzo TD Jr, eds. *Essentials of Physical Medicine and Rehabilitation.* Philadelphia, PA: Elsevier; 2015:chap 123:628.

Piper BF, Cella D. Cancer-related fatigue: definitions and clinical subtypes. *J Natl Compr Cancer Netw.* August 8, 2010;8:958-966.

CASE 4: HIV REHABILITATION

A 22-year-old man with HIV is referred to the PM&R clinic by his infectious disease specialist because of weakness and fatigue. He was diagnosed 4 years ago, and was started on HAART therapy. He has not been compliant with his regimen. His CD4 count last month was 250/mm (normal > 500/mm) and his viral load was 10,000 copies (normal undetectable).

Questions

1. What questions would you ask him to further delineate the cause of his weakness?

2. You learn his weakness is generalized and began about 1 month ago, and has been progressive. He reports muscle aches and fatigue. He has difficulty arising from a chair and climbing stairs. His knees buckle with prolonged standing or walking more than a block. He has lost about 5 kg (10 lbs) this month. He has no fevers, numbness, headaches, diplopia, dysphagia, or bowel or bladder incontinence. Vital signs are normal. What physical exam findings are important to illicit?

3. He has no cranial nerve deficits. He has muscle wasting and 4/5 strength in his proximal muscle; distally he is 5/5. Reflexes are normal. Sensation is intact. Range of motion is full in all four limbs and the spine. There is no vertebral tenderness. What is your differential diagnosis for his weakness? What diagnostic tests are indicated?

4. His CPK, ESR, and testosterone levels are normal. EMG/NCS shows normal NCS and low amplitude polyphasic MUPs without spontaneous activity. What treatment would you recommend?

5. At the conclusion of his visit with you, he complains of loss of libido. He would like you to prescribe sildenafil (Viagra). How should you respond?

6. He reports he can't afford his insurance copays for physical therapy. What are options for this?

CASE 4: HIV REHABILITATION

Answers

1. Ask about the course and timing of symptoms. Inquire about muscle pain, numbness, and functional limitations. Perform a complete review of systems (especially constitutional).

2. Look for muscle wasting and perform manual muscle testing. Check sensation and cranial nerves. Palpate for vertebral tenderness.

3. Differential diagnosis includes AIDS sarcopenia, polymyositis, polyneuropathy, and vertebral osteomyelitis. Testing should include CPK, ESR, testosterone level, and EMG/NCS.

4. He likely has AIDS sarcopenia. A resistive exercise program is the most effective treatment. Testosterone replacement is controversial in AIDS patients with normal testosterone levels; it does help increase muscle mass but balance this with side effects.

5. Sexuality should be addressed in a nonjudgmental way. Does the patient get morning erections? Is the issue loss of libido or erectile dysfunction? Engage the patient in a nonjudgmental discussion of the necessity of condom protection—does the patient perceive barriers to his compliance to this? Does he understand the implications for his sexual partners?

6. Usually charitable organizations will not help much for patients who have health insurance. He could do a home exercise program, with your instructions, and purchase dumbbells at a relatively low cost.

BIBLIOGRAPHY

Dudgeon WD, Phillips KD, Carson JA, et al. Counteracting muscle wasting in HIV infected individuals. *HIV Med.* 2006;7:299-310.

Levinson SF, Fine SM. Rehabilitation of patient with HIV. In: Fronterra W, ed. *Delisa's Physical Medicine and Rehabilitation: Principles and Practice.* 5th ed. Philadelphia, PA: Lippincott Williams & Wilkins; 2010:chap 47.

4 Cardiovascular and Pulmonary Rehabilitation

Matthew N. Bartels

CASE 1: CARDIAC REHABILITATION: INPATIENT

A 55-year-old man with a history of coronary artery disease starting a week ago when he was admitted for a myocardial infarction is now 5 days postoperative for a coronary bypass graft surgery. He had severe triple vessel disease and had a myocardial infarction followed by an attempted angioplasty, which was converted to an emergent surgery. He has just been sent from the ICU to the floor and rehabilitation assessment is obtained.

Questions

1. What information would you seek from the chart and what questions would you ask him to further delineate his case?

2. You learn he had four-vessel coronary disease with an LAD occlusion that could not be opened via angioplasty. Subsequently he had a median sternotomy with coronary artery bypass graft x4. He had a cross clamp time of 1 hour with a bypass time of 2.5 hours. The ICU course was notable for initial sedation, but he is now fully responsive and has been out of bed since postoperative day 1. By report he has had a relatively uncomplicated operative course otherwise. Asking him how he feels, you find that he has incisional pain, fatigue, mild shortness of breath, and loss of appetite. He has no focal neurologic symptoms. What will you look for on physical exam?

3. His exam is notable for a mild sternal click on cough and he has palpable motion with movement. There are decreased breath sounds at the left lung base. There is mild erythema at the SVG donor sites, but no clear infection. He has stable blood pressure and no orthostasis. His EKG has no marked ectopy and he has evidence of an anterior wall infarction on the cardiogram. What further information will help you design an exercise program?

4. He has had a postoperative echocardiogram that shows he has an ejection fraction of 30% with anterior wall hypokinesis. Chest x-ray shows a mild to moderate layering left chest effusion. What treatment would you recommend? How will you know he is ready for discharge?

5. At the conclusion of his in-hospital mobilization, he is ready for discharge, walking independently and able to climb two flights of stairs independently without ectopy or dyspnea. He asks you what the next steps will be. What are your recommendations?

6. In lay terms, explain key components of secondary prevention.

CASE 1: CARDIAC REHABILITATION: INPATIENT

Answers

1. Presenting symptoms and findings, catheterization findings, intraoperative course, and ICU status (kidney function, recovery of neurologic status, ectopy, and arrhythmias).

2. The physical exam should focus on peripheral extremities, looking for evidence of heart failure, assessing SVG donor sites, sternal wound, and particularly sternal stability. Also to be assessed are his hemodynamics, including heart rate and pulses. Mental state and neurologic exam are also key. Assess for musculoskeletal or neurologic impairments of the lower limbs.

3. Assess the echocardiogram, chest x-ray (especially with left lung base dull), CBC to rule out infection, and EKG/telemetry data. Demonstrate that the sternal instability will be addressed with sternal precautions and discussed with the team (this could be a long-term issue), and that there is an awareness of congestive heart failure with damaged heart modifying the exercise program. There will also be a need to recognize that effusions are common postoperatively and need to be monitored at this level.

4. Thoracentesis or pericardiocentesis may be needed if the effusion increases in the future (1 in 2,000 cases). The goal for discharge is independent ambulation and ability to do about 3 to 4 METs of exercise. He needs to be independent with sit to stand and bed mobility without breaking sternal precautions. This is often more challenging than gait.

5. This is the time for a mobilization program at home with walking at a level of 3 to 4 METs. He should be referred for an outpatient cardiac rehabilitation program, which will need to start several weeks postdischarge. He will not be able to do full upper activities and will have sternal precautions for 6 weeks postsurgery. Finally, he will need to start secondary prevention, which can start immediately with education.

6. Using eighth-grade level language, go through the basics. Smoking cessation (if applicable) is a must. Weight loss is also essential. This is done through portion control and a diet low in sugar, starches, and saturated fat (the latter may need more explanation). Exercise as you've learned in your cardiac rehabilitation program is vital. If you have high blood pressure, you need to lower your salt intake and take your blood pressure medicine. You should also take medication to lower your cholesterol, and to slow your heart. A baby aspirin daily can be one of the simplest ways to lower risk.

BIBLIOGRAPHY

Bartels MN. Cardiopulmonary rehabilitation. In: Batmangelich S, ed. *Physical Medicine and Rehabilitation Patient Centered Care.* New York, NY: Demos Publishing; 2014:112-129.

Bartels MN, Prince DZ. Acute medical conditions. In: Cifu DX, ed. *Braddom's Physical Medicine and Rehabilitation.* 5th ed. Philadelphia, PA: Elsevier, Inc.; 2015:571-595.

CASE 2: CARDIAC REHABILITATION OUTPATIENT

A 60-year-old woman with no heart attack, but just treated with an angioplasty for single vessel coronary disease, is referred for outpatient cardiac rehabilitation. She is presenting for initial evaluation 3 days after the angioplasty.

Questions

1. What questions would you ask her to further delineate cardiac disease?

2. You learn of a significant family history with both parents affected and also an older brother. She has multiple lifestyle issues including obesity, smoking, sedentary lifestyle, and early menopause. What physical exam points would you look for?

3. She has cholesteatoma, and has severe arthritis in her knees. You find that she also has mild peripheral vascular disease with an ABI of 0.90. Her sensation is intact and her neurologic exam is normal. Cardiac exam is also normal. What diagnostic tests are indicated?

4. Why is it important to assess for lower limb impairments?

5. A review of her lab data shows a normal cardiogram and an echo-cardiogram with EF of 55%, normal valve function. Catheterization data shows single vessel occlusion of the circumflex with patent graft after bare metal stent. She has total cholesterol of 300 with LDL 180. BMI is 32.4, with normal blood chemistries and normal CBC. What treatment regimen would you recommend?

6. She will start cardiac rehabilitation and secondary prevention. You will enroll her in smoking cessation and a nutritionally guided weight loss program. However, the smoking and weight loss programs won't have openings for more than 1 month. How do you proceed with weight loss and smoking cessation?

7. She returns 1 month later, and has not stopped smoking and has not lost any weight. How would you counsel her?

CASE 2: CARDIAC REHABILITATION OUTPATIENT

Answers

1. Elicit full cardiac risk factors and history, including family history and possible comorbid conditions (stroke, peripheral vascular disease).

2. The examination needs to include chest/cardiac exam, peripheral vascular status, neurologic exam, and signs of stigmata of hypercholesterolemia.

3. Assess the cardiogram, echo (LVEF assessment), catheterization data, procedure review, and blood tests including a lipid profile and glycosylated hemoglobin.

4. She may require accommodations such as using cycle or upper limb ergometry in lieu of a treadmill.

5. Her obesity, smoking, and sedentary lifestyle are the major issues. She will need to have smoking cessation counseling, recommendation for nutritional assessment/treatment, start of an exercise program, and start of secondary prevention.

6. Smoking cessation and weight control will be the hardest secondary prevention issues and will need to be addressed together as many individuals who stop smoking gain weight. Starting the smoking cessation as soon as possible is essential, and assistance with abstinence can help with pharmacological interventions. This can be medications in combination with nicotine replacement as well as counseling. Counseling for nutrition should include portion control as well as avoidance of animal fats and processed carbohydrates.

7. Motivational interviewing has been shown to be more effective than lecturing. Assess her readiness to change. Ask her what the barriers are to smoking cessation and weight loss. Address these together by problem solving.

BIBLIOGRAPHY

Balady GJ, Williams MA, Ades PA, et al. Core components of cardiac rehabilitation/secondary prevention programs: 2007 update: a scientific statement from the American Heart Association Exercise, Cardiac Rehabilitation, and Prevention Committee, the Council on Clinical Cardiology; the Councils on Cardiovascular Nursing, Epidemiology and Prevention, and Nutrition, Physical Activity, and Metabolism; and the American Association of Cardiovascular and Pulmonary Rehabilitation. *Circulation.* May 22, 2007;115(20):2675-2682.

Bartels MN. Cardiopulmonary rehabilitation. In: Batmangelich S, ed. *Physical Medicine and Rehabilitation Patient Centered Care.* New York, NY: Demos Publishing; 2014:112-129.

Piepoli MF, Corra U, Adamopoulos S, et al. Secondary prevention in the clinical management of patients with cardiovascular diseases. Core components, standards and outcome measures for referral and delivery: a policy statement from the cardiac rehabilitation section of the European Association for Cardiovascular Prevention & Rehabilitation. Endorsed by the Committee for Practice Guidelines of the European Society of Cardiology. *European Journal of Preventive Cardiology.* June 2014;21(6):664-681.

CASE 3: VASCULAR REHABILITATION

A 67-year-old man with diabetes and a vague history of cardiac disease is referred to the PM&R clinic by his general internist because of claudication and gait difficulty. He was diagnosed with angina 4 years ago and treated medically with medications (beta blockade, aspirin, and nitrates). He was also started on antihyperlipidemics and told to improve his diabetic control, but he has not been as compliant with his regimen as could be desired. In addition, he has continued to smoke. He presents for evaluation.

Questions

1. What questions would you ask him to further delineate his vascular disease?

2. You learn his vascular symptoms include pain with walking for more than one block, and he has had no resting pain. He does state that his feet are numb and he has more difficulty with walking up hills and walking quickly. What physical exam findings are important to illicit?

3. He has no ulcerations, but has absent pulses and has trophic skin changes. He has decreased sensation and also has foot fungus at the toenails with poor toenail hygiene. What further physical tests will you do on his exam?

4. His ankle-brachial index (ABI) is 0.55. What further evaluation will you order?

5. His blood tests reveal elevated cholesterol with an elevated LDL, elevated HgA1c, and normal ESR and CBC. EKG shows evidence of an old inferior wall myocardial infarction and normal sinus rhythm. What treatment would you recommend?

6. What exercise prescription will you give? What medications would you recommend?

7. At the conclusion of his visit with you, he complains of loss of erectile function. He would like you to prescribe sildenafil (Viagra). How should you respond?

8. Secondary prevention is critical for this patient. What other things should he be mindful about, and what other health care professionals might be enlisted?

CASE 3: VASCULAR REHABILITATION

Answers

1. Ask about the course/timing of symptoms; leg/resting pain; numbness; functional limitations; chest pain and shortness of breath; and perform a complete review of systems (also consider a neurologic exam as stroke is a comorbid condition).

2. In the physical exam, check for muscle wasting, manual muscle testing, sensation, blood pressure, cardiac exam, peripheral pulses, and skin exam.

3. Consider ankle-brachial indices (ABI), a test to be done in the office. You could also do a step test or 6 minute walk test as field screening tests. Differential: peripheral vascular disease, peripheral neuropathy (diabetic), vascular insufficiency, comorbid cardiac ischemic disease, comorbid COPD.

4. Lab work should include lipid profile, HbA1C, CBC, ESR, and ECG.

5. He has significant PVD and also has evidence of old MI. This will complicate his treatment regimen as he will be at risk of ischemia with mobilization. Exercise therapy is recommended, as well as smoking cessation and secondary prevention with education, lifestyle modification, and diabetic teaching.

6. Exercise will include aerobic training focused on ambulation. Heart rate precautions will be 20 BPM above resting heart rate (on beta-blocker) if no CPET can be arranged. Strengthening exercises as well as postural and balance training will be appropriate. He will benefit from cardiac evaluation only if not recently done. Monitoring will be optional, but nice if available.

7. Sexuality should be addressed. He likely has significant vascular disease that is causing impotence. Does the patient get morning erections? If none, and there is vascular erectile dysfunction in the setting of nitrates, he cannot start to use Viagra. This should be addressed with the patient. Referral to urology for alternative erectile dysfunction treatment methods is warranted.

8. He is at risk for foot ulcers and amputation. He should be trained to monitor his feet, and may need a podiatrist. He should have regular eye exams for retinopathy. He is at risk for coronary disease, and should be instructed about signs and symptoms of angina.

BIBLIOGRAPHY

Hamburg NM, Balady GJ. Exercise rehabilitation in peripheral artery disease: functional impact and mechanisms of benefits. *Circulation.* 2011;123:87-97.

Peripheral Arterial Disease Exercise Training Toolkit. AACVPR resources. Available at: http://www.vascularcures.org/images/PDFDiseases-Flyers/focus-onwalkingflyer.pdf

Writing Committee to Develop Guidelines for the Management of Patients With Peripheral Arterial Disease. ACC/AHA guidelines for the management of patients with peripheral arterial disease (lower extremity, renal, mesenteric, and abdominal aortic): executive summary: a collaborative report from the American Association for Vascular Surgery/Society for Vascular Surgery, Society for Cardiovascular Angiography and Interventions, Society for Vascular Medicine and Biology, Society of Interventional Radiology, and the ACC/AHA Task Force on Practice Guidelines. *J Am Coll Cardiol.* 2006;1:1-17.

CASE 4: PULMONARY REHABILITATION

A 68-year-old man with a 40 pack year history of smoking with severe respiratory failure was admitted to the ICU and intubated. He is now seeing you for rehabilitation.

Questions

1. What are the rehabilitation issues for this intubated individual? He is currently awake on the ventilator, but unable to be weaned. How would you proceed with assessment?

2. He has a history of smoking and was otherwise well until his admission. He has no clear history of cardiac disease and has been stable with respect to cardiac disease. You obtain a history and perform an exam that shows no clear neurologic deficits. He is very thin, but has good strength on individual muscle testing. Lung exam shows much reduced breath sounds. He has hyperreflexia and tachycardia with normal blood pressure. How will you start mobilization in the ICU?

3. After successful early mobilization, he is able to be extubated hospital day 6 and is discharged to the ward on hospital day 7. He is now starting mobilization on the floor. What are your next steps?

4. He is treated with antibiotics and steroids and started on a stable inhaler regimen. He has mild oxygen desaturation with exertion, and is controlled in therapy with supplemental oxygen, 1 liter via nasal cannula at rest and 2 liters with activity. On hospital day 9 he is ready for discharge. What are your plans?

5. Pulmonary function tests reveal severe obstructive disease with hyperinflation and no bronchodilator response. He now presents to your outpatient pulmonary rehabilitation program. What are the baseline assessments you will need for his pulmonary rehabilitation program?

6. He now is enrolled in the program. What are your goals and precautions in the rehabilitation program?

7. He has not stopped smoking. How could you counsel him effectively?

8. What are key elements in developing an ICU rehab consult service?

CASE 4: PULMONARY REHABILITATION

Answers

1. Prevention of the complications of immobility needs to be addressed (deep vein thrombosis, skin, urinary tract infection, pulmonary) as well as starting early mobilization. There is also the need for you to complete an assessment of strength and mental status, which can be done on the ventilator. Also gather data about the patient's condition, based on chest x-ray and ventilator settings.

2. Hyperreflexia may reflect beta agonists and not relate to neurologic deficits in this population; the same is true with tachycardia. He has good strength despite cachexia, which is also a finding in this group of patients. Recognizing he is stable, the plan should be for early mobilization of the patient, even while on the ventilator.

3. After starting early mobilization, the patient needs follow-up on the floor. He has no history of pulmonary rehabilitation and needs to start with goals of education and secondary prevention along with medication education, as well as disease management and oxygen use education. He needs a full assessment of his pulmonary and physical status as well, now that he is out of the ICU and off the ventilator.

4. Starting appropriate supplemental oxygen is essential. The goal is keeping saturation above a minimum of 90%. Low flow oxygen is also essential for a patient with COPD. One should closely monitor the pulse oximetry during increased levels of activity and adjust oxygen flow rates accordingly. Inhaled medications are essential to managing COPD, and pulmonary rehabilitation has a major role in educating patients about the medications and the proper administration of the inhalers (many patients cannot do it well).

5. You will need chest imaging and an exercise test (6 minute walk or shuttle at the low end, ideally a cardiopulmonary exercise test [CPET]). EKG and cardiac assessment in selected patients are appropriate, and an arterial blood gas (ABG) can also be useful if there is drowsiness or other sedation (may be hypercarbic on the supplemental oxygen or hypoxemic).

6. Goals are secondary prevention, family and patient education, home exercise program, and a pulmonary rehabilitation program with strengthening and conditioning. Monitoring will be for vital signs and O_2 saturation. Precautions include heart rate and blood pressure (especially diastolic ceilings), as well as maintaining oxygen saturation above 90%. Finally, medication education and training in inhalers and oxygen management need to be done.

7. Motivational interviewing is a well-documented, effective approach. You should ask him about readiness to change his habit, barriers to doing so, and how he perceives he could successfully overcome those barriers. The approach is nonjudgmental, and uses adult learning approaches to patient education.

8. Familiarize yourself with the scientific literature that supports early mobilization in the ICU to reduce mortality, morbidity, and costs. Engage the ICU physicians in this. Work with hospital administration to assign physical therapists to the ICU, and educate the therapists regarding the feasibility of getting patients to exercise and mobilize while still ventilated. Establish guidelines for safe mobilization in terms of cardiopulmonary stability.

BIBLIOGRAPHY

Bartels MN. Cardiopulmonary rehabilitation. In: Batmangelich S, ed. *Physical Medicine and Rehabilitation Patient Centered Care.* New York, NY: Demos Publishing; 2014:112-129.

Bartels MN, Prince DZ. Acute medical conditions. In: Cifu DX, ed. *Braddom's Physical Medicine and Rehabilitation.* 5th ed. Philadelphia, PA: Elsevier, Inc.; 2015:571-595.

Cameron S, Ball I, Cepinskas G, et al. Early mobilization in the critical care unit: a review of adult and pediatric literature [Review]. *J Crit Care.* August 2015;30(4):664-672.

Kruis AL, Smidt N, Assendelft WJ, et al. Integrated disease management interventions for patients with chronic obstructive pulmonary disease [Review]. *Cochrane Database Syst Rev.* 2013;10:CD009437.

Durable Medical Equipment

Brad E. Dicianno

A 34-year-old woman with lumbar level myelomeningocele presents for an assistive technology evaluation. She is complaining of recurrent skin breakdown and is worried it is related to her wheelchair.

Questions

1. What key elements about her history would you need to elicit?

2. She uses a power wheelchair that is 2 years old and which has had minor repair issues. She has tilt, recline, elevating leg rests, and a foam cushion. She does not use the seat functions regularly. She is on a bladder catheterization program and rarely incontinent of urine, but occasionally incontinent of bowel. Nutrition is good with adequate protein. She says that her transfers and pressure relief maneuvers are becoming difficult to conduct independently because of shoulder pain. She thinks this is contributing to some shear when she is transferring. What key physical exam findings would you want to collect?

3. She required minimum assistance to transfer out of the wheelchair onto a mat table. She has a 2-cm, Stage II pressure ulcer on her right ischial tuberosity, with moderate serosanguineous drainage and clean borders. Stool incontinence is present. She had no appreciable scoliosis on her exam. She has 2/5 strength in the bilateral hip flexors but otherwise 0/5 strength in lower limbs. She has absent sensation in the L2 dermatome and below bilaterally. What is the differential diagnosis for the skin breakdown?

4. What type of testing would you want to order?

5. Pressure mapping shows a significantly elevated area of pressure under the right ischial tuberosity. Besides appropriate wound care, what other interventions would you propose to help heal the pressure sore?

6. What education should be provided to this patient?

7. What social issues are important to consider in this case?

8. A physical therapist in your clinic wants to begin a quality improvement (QI) project. Discuss how you might implement a QI project that uses assistive technology and addresses skin breakdown.

9. You learn that due to the patient's cognitive impairment, she has had difficulty in the past with keeping an air cushion properly inflated. What ethical considerations are to be made when selecting a new cushion for her?

CASE 1: WHEELCHAIR SEATING

Answers

1. Obtain information about the type of wheelchair she uses (manual, power assist, or power), and, if she uses a power wheelchair, whether she currently has and uses any power seat functions. Also ask whether she can transfer or conduct pressure relief maneuvers independently. It would also be useful to know what type of cushion she uses. Ask the age of the equipment and whether it is in disrepair. Obtain review of system data regarding incontinence/moisture, nutrition status, and any potential sources of pressure and shear.

2. On her exam, determine the size, stage, location, and condition of any skin breakdown. Evaluate her ability to transfer in and out of the equipment. Evaluate her seating position to determine if scoliosis or any other factors might be contributing to seating asymmetries. Evaluate her sensation and motor function in the lower limbs.

3. The etiology is possibly multifactorial, from a combination of pressure, shear, and incontinence.

4. Pressure mapping should be ordered.

5. A new cushion is likely indicated, and ideally the selection of a cushion may depend on which demo cushion showed the best pressure distribution on pressure mapping. Generally, air or gel cushions provide better pressure relief than foam cushions. Tilt, combined with recline, offer the best pressure relief for this type of wound. The physiatrist should work with the therapist to determine if changes can be made to her seating positioning to reduce asymmetry in seating that might be causing more pressure on the right side. She would also benefit from a better bowel program to improve incontinence.

6. She will require education on risk for skin breakdown and the fact that the causes are multifactorial. She will require education on the proper use of power seat functions. Transfer training may be warranted. Education about pressure and shear on other surfaces such as commodes or shower chairs may also be warranted.

7. Her living situation, availability of caregivers, financial resources, insurance coverage, and ability to transport her wheelchair may provide insight into barriers to independence and mobility.

8. Some options might be instituting a comprehensive screening for all etiologies of skin breakdown, implementing evidence-based practice guidelines on the prevention and treatment of skin breakdown, or a patient education program. You would need to establish outcome measures, such as the frequency of pressure sores, and then track whether the intervention affected this outcome.

9. First, "do no harm." The principle of nonmaleficence is appropriate to apply here. Although an air cushion might provide good pressure relief, it might be difficult to maintain, and therefore cause harm to the patient. Choose a cushion that provides good pressure relief but is also easy for her to maintain.

BIBLIOGRAPHY

Cooper RA. Wheelchair adjustment and maintenance. In: Cooper RA, ed. *Wheelchair Selection and Configuration.* New York, NY: Demos Medical Publishing;1998:371-390.

Dicianno BE, Lieberman J, Schmeler MR, et al. Rehabilitation engineering and assistive technology society of North America's position on the application of tilt, recline, and elevating legrests for wheelchairs literature update. *Assist Technol.* 2015;27(3):193-198. Available at: https://www.medicare.gov/coverage/durable-medical-equipment -coverage.html

Dicianno BE, Schmeler M, Liu B. Wheelchairs/adaptive mobility equipment and seating. In: Campagnolo DI, Kirshblum S, Nash MS, et al., eds. *Spinal Cord Medicine.* 2nd ed. Philadelphia, PA: Lippincott Williams & Wilkins; 2012:341-358.

CASE 2: STROKE

A 78-year-old, right-handed man with a right middle cerebral artery stroke and left hemiparesis presents for an assistive technology evaluation. He completed inpatient and outpatient rehabilitation but has not regained ambulation ability that is sufficient for him to be able to complete activities of daily living inside the home, and he is not able to go out into the community due to fear of falling.

Questions

1. What key elements about his history would you need to elicit?

2. He was discharged from inpatient rehabilitation with a rented fold-ing lightweight manual wheelchair with adjustable tension backrest, standard foam cushion, and removable leg rests. He cannot push it because of his hemiparesis. He uses a wheeled walker and an ankle foot orthosis when he ambulates. He can ambulate and transfer independently but describes his walking as slow. He denies signifi-cant spasticity or falls. He has some mild left shoulder pain. He does not have a wheelchair of his own. He wants a device that is easily transportable. He lives with his wife, and they have a small compact car. He is retired and wants to spend time with his grandchildren. They live in an apartment that has two steps to enter and cannot be ramped. What key physical exam findings would you want to collect?

3. He has normal strength in the right hemibody. On the left side he has pain with testing of the shoulder and deltoids are 2/5. Distally, his strength is 3/5. In the left lower limb, hip flexors are 2/5, quad-riceps 3, and dorsiflexors 2/5. Sensation is decreased on the left hemibody but normal on the right. Tone is MAS 1 in the left arm and leg. Range of motion is normal, but his left shoulder is sub-luxed. There is a mild left visual neglect. Transfers are modified independent with a walker. Gait is functionally slow and hemi-paretic with poor advancement of the left leg. The leg is slightly externally rotated when he advances it. Explain why the patient is having difficulty walking despite having an AFO and a walker.

4. What assistive technology intervention would be indicated for this patient?

5. What education should be provided to this patient?

6. The patient is concerned about insurance coverage for a wheel-chair. He has Medicare. Explain whether this device would be cov-ered by insurance.

CASE 2: STROKE

Answers

1. Obtain information about the type of assistive technology that he has used so far (e.g., wheelchair, assistive device such as a cane or crutch, orthoses). Ask about level of independence with transfers and ambulation. Obtain review of systems data regarding spasticity, falls, and pain. Obtain information about what type of technology he would like, employment status, and social history including his mode of transportation.

2. On his exam, evaluate strength, muscle tone, sensation, range of motion, gait, and transfers. Also evaluate for any visual neglect. Perform a thorough musculoskeletal examination of the shoulder.

3. Although the patient's foot drop is corrected with the brace, the patient has weak hip flexors that are causing problems advancing the leg. Additionally, spasticity, decreased sensation, and neglect may be contributing to impaired functional mobility. Shoulder pain may be causing difficulty with using the walker.

4. The best choice of equipment for this patient is likely a manual wheelchair with low seat height, which would allow for propulsion using one arm and leg.

5. He requires education on wheelchair skills and propulsion, wheelchair maintenance, and joint preservation.

6. Medicare Part B covers 80% of durable medical equipment such as wheelchairs.

BIBLIOGRAPHY

Cooper RA. Manual wheelchairs. In: Cooper RA, ed. *Wheelchair Selection and Configuration*. New York, NY: Demos Medical Publishing;1998:199-223.

CASE 3: AMBULATORY ASSISTIVE DEVICES

An 82-year-old female with end-stage right hip osteoarthritis presents to your clinic due to falls. She complains of right hip pain and tells you that she has not been interested in hip surgery due to her age and other comorbid conditions, including a prior myocardial infarction. She would like to know what she can do to prevent falls. She describes her balance as poor.

Questions

1. What key elements about her history would you need to elicit?

2. She describes her falls as being accompanied by pain and her hip "giving out." She denies losses of consciousness or tripping over objects. She uses a cane. She is right handed and prefers using the cane in that hand. She recently finished land-based and aquatic therapy, which improved pain, but she is still occasionally falling. Her medication list includes aspirin, a beta blocker, an antianxiety medication (lorazepam), and an anticholinergic medication for her bladder, but she says that she does not like to take medications and takes only acetaminophen. She denies any diabetes or loss of sensation. She recently had cataract surgery and describes her vision as "good." What key physical exam findings would you want to collect?

3. She has 4+ to 5/5 strength in the lower body, except for the right hip. Although pain inhibited, her strength in the right hip abductors and flexors is 4-. Sensation and muscle bulk are normal. Passive range of motion of her right hip is limited by pain, but her left hip range of motion is normal. During stance phase on the right, the left side of her pelvis tilts down, and her trunk leans to the right. Her gait is also antalgic on the right. Her elbow is flexed approximately 25° when using the cane. Explain why the patient is perceiving balance problems.

4. What suggestions do you have for her assistive device use?

5. She is reluctant to use a walker due to cosmetic considerations. How would you counsel her?

6. What instructions would you give to the physical therapist to strengthen the hip?

7. Propose a way you could screen patients for fall risk in your clinic.

CASE 3: AMBULATORY ASSISTIVE DEVICES

Answers

1. Obtain information about the nature of her falls (e.g., mechanical, syncope). Ask about assistive device use and assess whether the devices have been used properly. Enquire about any therapies received. Evaluate for other etiologies for falling, such as multiple medication usage, low vision, or peripheral neuropathy.

2. On exam, evaluate strength, muscle bulk, sensation, range of motion, and gait. Also evaluate for any visual impairments. Perform a thorough musculoskeletal examination of the hip.

3. The patient has a compensated Trendelenburg gait because of left hip abductor weakness. She is compensating for the drop in her pelvis with a trunk lean to the right. The antalgic gait on the right causes her to spend less time in stance phase on the right. Because she is using a cane on the antalgic side, she is also loading her right hip with unnecessary force during walking.

4. The cane seems to be at the proper height since the elbow is flexed between 20° to 30°, but should be switched to the left side to offload the right hip during ambulation. Physical therapy may be required to train her to use the cane properly or to trial a walker.

5. Be sensitive to her concerns and acknowledge them. Remind her of the risks of falling, and how a hip fracture or other injuries might impact her.

6. Although any type of resistance training can improve strength, isometric strength training is generally indicated in the presence of a painful joint because it is better tolerated.

7. Possible answers include using validated fall risk surveys or functional evaluations. To be cost and time effective, you may want to have your medical assistant ask these questions, or perhaps have patients complete a questionnaire while in the waiting area.

BIBLIOGRAPHY

Bennell KL, Dobson F, Hinman RS. Exercise in osteoarthritis: moving from prescription to adherence. *Best Pract Res Clin Rheumatol*. 2014;28(1):93-117.

Blount WP. Don't throw away the cane. *J Bone Joint Surg Am*. 1956;38-A(3):695-708.

Kumar R, Roe MC, Scremin OU. Methods for estimating the proper length of a cane. *Arch Phys Med Rehabil*. 1995;76(12):1173-1175.

CASE 4: LIGHTWEIGHT WHEELCHAIR PRESCRIPTION

A 22-year-old male with T9 AIS A spinal cord injury presents to your assistive technology clinic for a mobility device evaluation. His current manual wheelchair is in disrepair and he is interested in a wheelchair he saw on a website.

Questions

1. What key elements about his history would you need to elicit?

2. He currently uses a folding (cross-brace) manual wheelchair which is about 5 years old. He is able to transfer independently. He is employed as an accountant and drives an adapted vehicle. He wants to start playing wheelchair basketball and tennis (Figure 5.1). He has a prior rotator cuff tear that was repaired, but he has some residual right shoulder pain that does not limit activity. He has a remote history of a pressure ulcer on his sacrum but no recent skin breakdown. He is mostly continent of bowel and bladder when compliant with his bladder and bowel routines. What key physical exam findings would you want to collect?

3. He has 5/5 strength in the upper body and 0/5 strength in the lower body. He has increased tone in the legs. Sensory level is at T9. Trunk balance is fair. Contractures are noted at the knees, but passive shoulder range of motion is normal. His right shoulder exam is relatively normal. Skin is intact. Explain how choosing a wheelchair and setting it up properly can help to mitigate shoulder pain.

4. The patient asks you to explain the advantages of solid frame ultralight wheelchairs, compared to folding frames.

5. What effect does fore/aft axle position have on wheelchair propulsion?

6. This patient wants to participate in two different adaptive sports, basketball and tennis. Explain what technology he would need and how it might be funded.

CASE 4: LIGHTWEIGHT WHEELCHAIR PRESCRIPTION

Answers

1. Obtain information about his current wheelchair including frame type. Obtain a functional history to include transfer ability. Ask about social history including employment, transportation, and leisure activities. Conduct a thorough review of systems including history of shoulder pain, incontinence, and skin breakdown.

2. On exam, evaluate strength, muscle tone, trunk balance, sensation, range of motion, and transfer ability. Inspect skin for breakdown. Perform a thorough musculoskeletal examination of the shoulder.

3. Keeping the weight of the individual and the wheelchair minimized, teaching proper wheelchair propulsion technique, and proper setup of the wheelchair (including axle position) can help to mitigate shoulder pain.

4. Solid frames are available as cantilever or box designs. Because they are solid, efficiency of propulsion and durability are higher than with a folding frame. Although the frames do not fold, they have quick-release wheels, and the backrests can be folded down for ease of transportability.

5. A rearward axle reduces access to the push rim, promoting an "arc" style of propulsion, increasing the strokes required to travel a given distance, and thereby predisposing the user to repetitive strain injuries. A rearward axle, however, makes the chair more stable. A forward axle promotes propulsion using long, smooth strokes (semicircular pattern), reducing stroke frequency. Moving the axle forward allows the chair to tip backward more easily for wheelies.

6. A person's everyday wheelchair is not typically used for sports. Each sport has its own wheelchair design that is geared specifically for that sport. So ideally, this person would need to use both basketball and tennis wheelchairs. However, sports equipment is not covered under standard private medical insurance. (Some options however are available for those with Veterans Affairs coverage.) Typically individuals would need to self-pay or identify other private funding sources if they wanted their own sports equipment. However, it would be helpful to refer this patient to a local adaptive sports organization that can get him started in sports and that may have equipment that participants share.

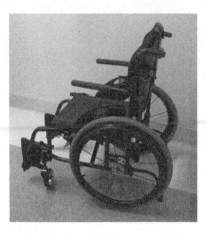

Figure 5.1 Lightweight active wheelchair.

BIBLIOGRAPHY

Cooper RA. Sports and alternative wheelchairs. In: Cooper RA, ed. *Wheelchair Selection and Configuration.* New York, NY: Demos Medical Publishing; 1998:271-290.

Dicianno B, Schmeler M, Liu B. Wheelchairs/adaptive mobility equipment and seating. In: Campagnolo DI, Kirshblum S, Nash MS, et al., eds. *Spinal Cord Medicine.* 2nd ed. Philadelphia, PA: Lippincott Williams & Wilkins; 2012:341-358. [VN12]

CASE 5: POWER MOBILITY DEVICES

A 52-year-old female with multiple sclerosis, diagnosed 6 months ago, presents to your assistive technology clinic for a mobility device evaluation. She has been using a depot (standard) manual wheelchair that she self-purchased, but she is having trouble propelling it because of upper limb weakness and fatigue. She is looking for a device to improve her mobility indoors and outdoors.

Questions

1. What key elements about this patient's history would you need to elicit?

2. She is able to walk independently with a left AFO and a walker, but gets fatigued after only a couple steps, which sometimes results in falls. She worked as a nurse's aide but is now unemployed. She would like to seek a different job. She was driving a compact car but stopped due to leg weakness. She enjoys traveling to visit her adult children and cooking. She lives with her husband in a small condominium. She has diffuse muscle cramps and admits to having a difficult time dealing with her diagnosis. What key physical exam findings would you want to collect?

3. She has 4/5 strength in the upper body, 2/5 strength in the left hip flexor and dorsiflexors, and 4/5 strength in the lower body otherwise. Tone is normal. Trunk balance is fair. Range of motion is normal. She needed assistance from her husband to transfer out of the wheelchair. Explain why the patient's transfer ability is important to consider when choosing a mobility device.

4. The patient asks about a scooter because she has used them in the past in the grocery store. What are the pros and cons of a scooter, compared to a power wheelchair, for this particular patient?

5. What other referrals might be indicated for this patient?

6. She is distraught about her progressive disability. How would you talk to her about this?

CASE 5: POWER MOBILITY DEVICES

Answers

1. Obtain information about her ability to walk and transfer, as well as assistive device use. Ask about social history including employment, living environment, transportation, and leisure activities. Conduct a thorough review of systems including history of pain and depressive symptoms.

2. On exam, conduct a musculoskeletal and neurologic exam to include strength, muscle tone, trunk balance, range of motion, and transfer ability.

3. If a person cannot transfer or weight shift independently, the person may be at risk for skin breakdown, and therefore may need a device with power seat functions that allow them to reposition independently.

4. Scooters (Figure 5.2) are sometimes viewed by patients as being more culturally acceptable, especially those newly adjusting to a diagnosis, and are less expensive than power wheelchairs. However, scooters have a wide turning radius that makes them less maneuverable in tight living spaces, can tip over on uneven surfaces, and require more strength to operate since they have a tiller. They also have no power features that assist weight shifting. A power wheelchair therefore is likely the better option for this patient.

5. This patient may benefit from being referred to vocational rehabilitation given her interest in seeking a different job, psychology to help her adjust to her disability, and to an adaptive driving program to determine whether she may be able to drive with adapted controls.

6. Acknowledge that multiple sclerosis can be particularly frustrating due to the unpredictability of prognosis. Most patients do well, and have slow progression, but some patients have more difficulty. Offer psychological consultation, referral for spiritual or religious guidance, and/or referral to patient support groups, many of which are available online.

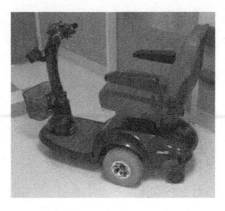

Figure 5.2 Power scooter.

BIBLIOGRAPHY

Cooper RA. Manual wheelchairs. In: Cooper RA, ed.*Wheelchair Selection and Configuration*. New York, NY: Demos Medical Publishing; 1998:199-223.

Dicianno BE, Lieberman J, Schmeler MR, et al. Rehabilitation engineering and assistive technology society of North America's position on the application of tilt, recline, and elevating legrests for wheelchairs literature update. *Assist Technol*. 2015;27(3):193-198. Available at: https://www.medicare.gov/coverage/durable-medical-equipment -coverage.html.

6 Geriatric Rehabilitation

George Forrest

An 80-year-old man is admitted to the hospital with community acquired pneumonia. He is treated with ceftriaxone and azithromycin. On the eighth day of the admission the hospitalist tells the patient that he has completed his course of antibiotics and he can go home. The patient tells the doctor "I do not think I am ready to go home. I feel very weak. I do not think that I can climb the stairs at the entrance to my home and I would not feel safe getting into and out of my tub." You are asked to evaluate the patient.

Questions

1. What would be important parts of the history that you obtain from the patient and from the patient's medical record?

2. The patient tells you that before he was admitted to the hospital he considered his health to be good for his age. He is living at home with his wife who is 78 and they had no help other than a woman who comes to help with cleaning once a week. He was not intubated or treated with steroids. He feels generally weak but he does not notice focal weakness or numbness. What would be important parts of the physical examination?

3. The patient's vital signs are normal. There is no drop in blood pressure when going supine to sit. The heart is regular, the lungs clear, abdomen benign, and no edema. The patient is alert and oriented. His responses to questions are all given with good logic and detail. His cranial nerve examination is normal. Reflexes are normal throughout all extremities. There is no alteration in tone or cogwheel rigidity. The patient moves all extremities through a full range of motion against gravity. You can very easily break his strength when he tries to maintain elevation of his shoulders. He has difficulty coming from sit to stand without rocking back and forth and pushing off with both hands. What likely has happened to impair this patient's transfers and function?

4. The patient tells you that he has been in the hospital for a week. During that time he did not feel well so he really got out of bed only to go to the bathroom. What are some of the physiologic changes that occur in patients who are on bed rest for a week?

5. What can be done to prevent this condition in future admissions?

6. His daughter expresses strong anger about her father having spent much of the last week in bed. How can you defuse her hostility?

CASE 1: ACUTE HOSPITAL CARE

Answers

1. You would want to know the patient's level of function prior to admission. You would want to know if the patient was intubated, was treated with steroids, or had positive blood cultures or multi-organ failure as these factors are associated with critical illness neuropathy/myopathy. You would want to know if the patient had any symptoms of a focal neurologic process such as a hemiplegia, sensory or motor level, or foot drop. You should ask about his home situation including environmental barriers and family support.

2. You would want to check the vital signs in particular, making sure that the fever has resolved and that the patient does not have orthostatic hypotension. You want to do a careful neurologic examination to make sure that there is no evidence of underlying Parkinson's disease, dementia, stroke, spinal cord injury, cerebellar disease, peroneal nerve injury, radiculopathy, or peripheral neuropathy. You should observe the patient doing bed mobility, transfers, and gait.

3. There are many possible causes of weakness in this patient. The list would include inflammatory muscle disease, connective tissue disease, vasculitis, hypothyroid or hyperthyroid disease, viral myositis, rhabdomyolysis, neuromuscular junction disease, paraneoplastic syndrome, hypokalemia, hypophosphatemia, low magnesium level, medications, demyelinating disease, radiculopathy, or medications. The history and examination do not suggest any of these problems. The most likely cause is weakness related to being in bed.

4. Muscle strength may decline by 1% to 1.5% per day. Antigravity muscles of the lower extremities are affected more than muscles of the upper extremities. Patients on bed rest lose 1% of bone mass of the vertebrae per week of bed rest. Patients on bed rest have a decrease in plasma volume. This results in increased heart rate at rest and, with activity, decreased stroke volume and orthostatic hypotension. Bed rest is associated with coagulopathy and increased risk of venous thrombosis, as well as increased insulin resistance, glucose intolerance, atelectasis, impaired respiratory function, and predisposition to pneumonia.

5. Studies show that giving patients exercises to do in bed, encouraging patients to get out of bed, and providing active therapies prevent the development of disuse atrophy. You could initiate a quality improvement project to encourage nursing and therapy staff to do this.

6. Express understanding and acknowledge her feelings. Do not lay blame on other team members, but offer to reinforce the importance of mobility with them. She should be referred to Patient Relations as well.

BIBLIOGRAPHY

Parry SM, Puthucheary ZA. The impact of extended bed rest on the musculoskeletal system in the critical care environment. *Extrem Physiol Med*. 2015;4:16. doi:10.1186/s13728-015-0035-7.

Topp R, Ditmyer M, King K, et al. The effect of bed rest and the potential of prehabilitation on patients in the intensive care unit. *AACN Clin Issues*. 2002;13(2):263-276.

CASE 2: GAIT DISTURBANCE

A 77-year-old man presents to your office and reports that he feels generally well but he is having some problems walking over the last few months. He has trouble getting up from his chair and his gait has slowed down. When he goes for walks with his wife he has trouble keeping up with her.

Questions

1. In the history and review of systems, what type of information would you be looking for?

2. Knowing the list of problems that might cause the patient's problem, what would you look for on physical examination?

3. The patient's vital signs are normal. There has been no loss of weight. Examination of the heart, lungs, and extremities is normal. The patient has no evidence of cognitive problems. The patient's tone and reflexes are normal. He can move all extremities well against gravity but you can easily break his hip flexors and knee extensors. Sensory examination is normal. You perform a get up and go test. You notice that the patient needs to use both hands to push off to get up and his time is 15 seconds, which is 3 seconds beyond the upper limit of normal. What is the differential diagnosis? What laboratory and diagnostic tests will you order?

4. All laboratory studies and the electrodiagnostic tests are normal. The patient takes no medications. What do you think explains the problems that the patient has described to you?

5. What advice can you give to the patient to retard the progression of his disease?

6. His wife expresses concern about the possibility of his falling. How might this be addressed in the home environment?

7. Explain the concept of sarcopenia in lay terms to the patient and his wife.

CASE 2: GAIT DISTURBANCE

Answers

1. Difficulty with strength and mobility can be symptoms of many types of medical problems. Start by asking why the patient is having difficulty walking. Is he short of breath, does he have fatigue, do his knees buckle, or does he have pain?

2. You always want to check vital signs including weight. You should check for orthostatic hypotension. You want to listen to the heart and lungs and check the extremities; look for signs of asthma, COPD, congestive heart failure, or arrhythmia. You want to check for muscle atrophy or muscle tenderness and examine large and small joints. You want to do a full neurologic examination including mental status, cranial nerves, tone, reflexes, strength, sensation, and gait.

3. The most important differential diagnoses in an elderly man with proximal weakness and normal reflexes and sensation are sarcopenia, myopathy, hypothyroidism, polymyalgia rheumatica, motor neuron disease, adrenal insufficiency, occult malignancy, and anemia. Considering the differential diagnoses you order a CBC, chemistry profile, thyroid function tests, C reactive protein or sedimentation rate, CPK, vitamin D level, and an EMG/NCV.

4. The disorder most consistent with the patient's presentation is sarcopenia. This is a loss of muscle strength that occurs in 14% of patients between 65 and 70 years of age and in slightly more than half of patients over 80 years of age. Manifestations are reduced grip strength, difficulty getting up from the seated position, impaired balance, and slow gait (<1.2 m/sec). Patients with sarcopenia have increased risk of falls and increased mortality.

5. Patients should be advised to perform one half hour of walking or stationary cycling per day if possible. Patients should be advised that people of any age can benefit from an appropriate program of resistance training. Patients should be told that it is important to have adequate protein intake, at least 1.3 g/kg/day. Patients should be checked for vitamin D deficiency and, if necessary, be given 880 IU per day as a supplement.

6. Environmental barriers such as clutter, excess furniture, and obstacles on the floor should be minimized. Night lights can be helpful. Grab bars in the bathroom are also important.

7. The examiner will be looking to you to use language at no more than the eighth grade level; avoid words with more than three syllables. Reiterate how aging causes a loss of muscle fibers and strength.

BIBLIOGRAPHY

Forrest G, Schott Z, Radu G. Geriatric gait and balance disorders. 2013. Available at: https://now.aapmr.org/?s=Forrest
+G%2C+Schott+Z%2C+Radu+G.+Geriatric+gait+and+balance+disorders

Saguil A. Evaluation of the patient with muscle weakness. *Am Fam Physician.* 2005;71(7):1327-1336.

Salzman B. Gait and balance disorders in older adults. *Am Fam Physician.* 2010;82:61-68.

Snijders AH, Van de Warrenburg BP, Giladi N, Bloem BR. Neurological gait disorders in elderly people: clinical approach and classification. *Lancet Neurol.* 2007;6:63-74.

Sudarsky L. Geriatrics: gait disorders in the elderly. *N Engl J Med.* 1990;322:1441-1446.

CASE 3: FALL PREVENTION

A 70-year-old woman comes to the office with her daughter. The daughter tells you that she is worried about her mom. "Mom feels well. She never complains but she just doesn't look steady on her feet. I am afraid she is going to fall."

Questions

1. What questions would you ask the patient?

2. The patient tells you that she has noticed that her gait is slower. She has not fallen but she just does not feel as steady as she used to. She is not sure why. She feels well. She does not take any medicines except for atorvastatin and amlodipine. She never feels as if she is going to black out and never has any sense of dizziness or spinning. She does not feel weak and has no numbness. Her friends all have problems with their backs or joints but she is lucky she does not have those problems. Describe the key portions of your examination.

3. What special tests could you do in the office or ask the physical therapist you work with to perform to help assess the risk that the patient might fall?

4. The patient's vital signs are normal and there is no orthostatic hypotension. Examinations of the heart, lungs, abdomen, and extremities are normal. Score on the Mini-Mental Status Exam is 30. The patient's vision is 20/30. She has some trouble hearing you when you whisper. Tone, reflexes, and manual muscle tests are normal. The patient has no difficulty distinguishing sharp from dull but proprioception seems mildly impaired. The patient can feel a tuning fork but when she no longer feels it on her foot you can feel it on your hand. There is no past pointing, and alternating movements do not show dysdiadochokinesia. The patient's gait has a normal heel to toe pattern and appears stable but the Romberg's test shows some sway when standing with the eyes closed. What do you think is wrong with the patient? What laboratory and diagnostic tests might you request?

5. How might this be addressed in the home environment?

6. The daughter asks if a home health agency could do a home safety evaluation. However, the patient is not homebound. Explain to her why Medicare will not cover this service.

CASE 3: FALL PREVENTION

Answers

1. You would ask the patient if she has fallen or if she is afraid of falling or if she has noticed a change in her gait. You would obtain a full history of her medical problems and ask which medications she takes. You would do a full review of systems, in particular wanting to know if there are symptoms of dizziness at rest, with change in position, or when coming from supine to sit or sit to stand. You would want to know about palpitations or history of arrhythmias. You would want to know about change in vision, hearing, or tinnitus. You would want to know if there was any history of focal weakness or numbness or if the patient noted any change in muscle tone, strength, or balance. You would want to know if she had any painful conditions suggestive of a radiculopathy or problems with her joints or her feet.

2. You check her vital signs including a check for orthostatic hypotension. You listen to her heart, checking for arrhythmia. You evaluate her joints and spine for range of motion and examine her feet. You perform a cognitive evaluation such as the Mini-Mental Status Exam or the Montreal Cognitive Assessment Test. You check the patient's vision with an eye card. You check hearing by the patient's ability to hear a whispered voice, watch, or tuning fork at about 2 feet from the ear. You check the patient's tone looking for rigidity or cog wheeling. You check reflexes and perform a manual muscle test of all four extremities. You check appreciation of light touch and pin prick. You check finger-nose-finger, alternating hand movements, and heel to shin testing. You check proprioception of the toes and vibration sense in the feet. You perform a Romberg's test and you watch the patient walk.

3. Two tests that can easily be performed in the office are the timed up and go test and the functional reach test. In the timed up and go test, the patient is asked to get up from a chair, walk 3 meters, and walk back to the chair and sit down. Ten seconds is considered a normal time and patients with a time of more than 14 seconds are considered at risk of fall. In the functional reach test the patient stands with feet shoulder-width apart. The patient raises one arm to 90° of flexion and is asked to reach forward without taking a step. Most patients can extend the third metacarpal at least 10 inches forward. A score of 6 to 7 inches is considered indicative of impaired balance. The Berg balance test is more time consuming. The patient is asked to perform 14 different maneuvers; each one is graded 0 to 4. The maneuvers are:
   (1) sit to stand;
   (2) standing to sitting;
   (3) placing a foot on a stool;
   (4) stand unsupported
   (5) reaching forward;
   (6) standing one foot in front of the other;
   (7) sit unsupported;
   (8) retrieving object from floor;
   (9) standing on one foot;
   (10) standing with eyes closed;

(11) looking over shoulder;
(12) transfer chair to chair;
(13) standing with feet together; and
(14) turning 360°.

A score of more than 40 is considered a low risk for fall; 21 to 40, a moderate risk for fall; and 0 to 20 a high risk for fall.

4. The history and examination do not suggest a problem with the heart or orthostasis. There are no symptoms or signs of vestibular disease, arthritis, or other musculoskeletal problems. There is not an indication of stroke, myelopathy, myopathy, or Parkinson's disease. The most common reason that a 70-year-old person would have difficulty with gait is age-related decline in the function of three systems involved with regulation of balance. These are vestibular, vision, and proprioception. The patient has impaired proprioception and appreciation of vibration and a positive Romberg's test. An EMG/NCV to evaluate for peripheral neuropathy would be helpful. A basic set of laboratory studies to investigate for peripheral neuropathy might include hemoglobin A1C, chemistry profile including fasting blood sugar, creatinine and liver function tests, vitamin B_{12}, thyroid function tests, erythrocyte sedimentation rate, SPEP, and ANA. Albumin can help assess nutritional status. Vitamin D deficiency is associated with muscle weakness and increased risk of fall. Additional tests that might be ordered in some patients depending upon the history include HIV serology, rheumatoid factor, Sjogren's syndrome testing (anti-Ro, anti-La antibodies), anti-Lyme antibodies, vitamin B_1, and hepatitis panel. This patient takes atorvastatin so a CPK might be helpful.

5. Studies have shown that exercise programs to improve strength, balance, and endurance can reduce the rate of falls. Recommendations for home safety include making sure that there is proper lighting and that there are railings on all staircases. Walking surfaces should provide good footing (eliminate shag rugs, throw rugs, electrical cords, and clutter). Grab bars and hand rails should be installed in the bathroom to increase safety during toileting and washing. The kitchen and bedrooms should be arranged to minimize the need for reaching and climbing.

6. Medicare does not cover therapies at home for patients who are not homebound. Furthermore, they will not cover occupational therapy as a sole service. Give her the facts about what Medicare will and will not cover. She may have the option to pay out of pocket for this service. Politely explain that you have no control over Medicare regulations, but you will do your best to advocate for services for which her mother does qualify.

BIBLIOGRAPHY

Berg K, Wood-Dauphinee S, Williams JI. The Balance Scale: reliability assessment with elderly residents and patients with an acute stroke. *Scand J Rehabil Med.* March 1995;27(1):27-36.

Lupsa BC, Insogna K. Bone health and osteoporosis. *Endocrinol Metab Clin North Am.* 2015;44:517-530.

Stubbs B, Denkinger MD, Brefka S, Dallmeier D. What works to prevent falls in community-dwelling older adults? Umbrella review of meta-analyses of randomized controlled trials. *Phys Ther.* August 2015;95(8):1095-1110. doi:10.2522/ptj.20140461.

Thomas GJ. Falls prevention in the elderly. *Knowledge Now.* Available at: http://me.aapmr.org/kn/article.html?id=77.

CASE 4: FITNESS

An older man comes to the office with his wife. The wife tells you, "Doctor, would you please try to put some sense into my husband's head? He is 82 years old. All of a sudden he wants to spend $600 to join a gym and start working out. Is this something that is necessary for an 82-year-old man?"

Questions

1. They ask you, "What are the recommendations for exercise for an 82-year-old man?"

2. The patient's wife asks you, "I understand the need for walking every day but why does he need to lift weights?" The wife adds, "He doesn't need to look better for me and I hope he is not trying to impress other women."

3. The patient says, "Doctor, thanks for the information. I was wondering if I need to get a stress test before I start the program?"

4. The wife asks you, "Doctor, what about his joints? Won't this program give him arthritis?"

5. The wife asks you, "Okay, Doctor. You have convinced me to let my husband join the fitness center. If we get a family membership what can I do? I have rheumatoid arthritis. My joints are really bad and I am not exactly skinny."

6. Explain to the wife in lay terms how exercise can benefit her.

CASE 4: FITNESS

Answers

1. A consensus panel from the American College of Sports Medicine and the American Heart Association recommends that patients of any age exercise for 30 minutes every day if possible. The program should include exercise to improve flexibility and aerobic exercise every day. Muscle strengthening exercises should be performed two or three days per week. Exercise sessions should begin with stretching and warm-up. Stretching should include static stretch to the muscles of the chest wall, hip flexors, hamstrings, and gastrocnemius muscles. Each group should have a static stretch of 15 to 30 seconds that is repeated three times on each side of the body. Warm-up consists of beginning the cardiovascular activity such as walking, jogging, biking, or swimming at a slow pace before beginning the aerobic exercise session. Moderate exercise is defined as being at 60% to 80% of maximum heart rate or VO_2 maximum, but it may be easier for patients to monitor their perceived level of exertion. If a person rates his or her level of exertion on a scale of 1 to 10, a rating of 5 or 6 corresponds to moderate activity; a rating of 7 or 8 corresponds to vigorous activity. Seniors may use the "talk test," which means that the participant is not too out of breath to comfortably talk. The aerobic session should end with a cool down period that is similar to the warm-up period. Strengthening activities should be done two or three nonconsecutive days per week. The participant should rate the exertion as 5 or 6 on a 10-point scale. It is recommended that 8 to 10 muscle groups are exercised. The weights used should be light enough that the participant can do 10 to 15 repetitions of each exercise. Weight-bearing calisthenics can be substituted for weight lifting. Exercise to improve balance is recommended but there are no specific recommendations as to which exercises should be done nor are there recommended protocols.

2. Muscle strength declines by 15% per decade after age 50 and by 30% per decade after age 70. Weight training can reduce or prevent the decline in strength that occurs with aging. The improved strength that occurs with exercise reduces the risk of fall in senior citizens. You would think that weight lifting would make you heavier by increasing muscle mass but it actually prevents obesity by improving insulin sensitivity and increasing metabolic rate by up to 15%. Weight training retards the osteoporosis that is associated with aging and it is associated with improved self-image and reduced incidence of depression.

3. The American College of Sports Medicine recommends a stress test for:
   • Men over age 45 and women over age 55 who plan to exercise at 60% of VO_2 maximum
   • Anyone with symptoms of cardiac disease or known cardiac disease
   • Anyone with signs or symptoms of pulmonary disease
   • Anyone with diabetes
   • Anyone with two or more risk factors for cardiac disease

If this patient has no history of cardiac disease and wants to begin his program with walking and very low resistance exercises such as lifting cans of soup, a stress test may not be necessary. For more vigorous exercise it would be prudent.

4. Contact sports or sports such as soccer in which there are frequent changes in direction that lead to acute knee injuries may be associated with development of degenerative changes in the knee but walking, jogging, cycling, and swimming are not associated with development of osteoarthritis and may be protective by improving the strength of the muscles that support the joints.

5. A program of flexibility training, low impact aerobic exercise, and low resistance muscle strengthening exercise is recommended for patents with rheumatoid arthritis. Patients who cannot tolerate the impact of walking or weight training may try to substitute cycling, aquatic therapy, and isometric exercises.

6. You should explain the benefits of weight control, pain control, cardiovascular conditioning, minimizing osteoporosis, and fall prevention. Illicit whether these are important to her. Ask her about barriers to participation.

BIBLIOGRAPHY

Fiatarone MA, O'Neill EF, Ryan ND, Clements KM, Solares GR, Nelson ME, Roberts SB, Kehayias JJ, Lipsitz LA, Evans WJ. Exercise training and nutritional supplementation for physical frailty in very elderly people. *N Engl J Med*. 1994 Jun 23;330(25):1769-75.

Metsios GS, Stavropoulos-Kalinoglou A, Kitas GD.The role of exercise in the management of rheumatoid arthritis. *Expert Rev Clin Immunol*. 2015;11(10):1121-30. doi:10.1586/1744666X.2015.1067606. Epub 2015 Jul 15. Review. PMID: 26178249

Neid RJ, Franklin B. Promoting and prescribing exercise for the elderly. *Am Fam Physician*. 2002;65:419-426.

Nelson ME, Rejeski WJ, Blair SN, et al. Physical activity and public health in older adults: recommendation from the American College of Sports Medicine and the American Heart Association. *Circulation*. 2007;116:1094-1105.

7 Musculoskeletal Impairments and Sports Medicine

Brian J. Krabak, Stephen Johnson, Brian C. Liem, Melinda S. Loveless, and Michael Mallow

CASE 1: SHOULDER PAIN IN MIDDLE AGE

A 53-year-old woman presents with a 6 month history of left shoulder pain and limited range of motion. She has never had this pain before and it is interfering with her daily activities.

Questions

1. What key elements do you want to know from her history?

2. She tells you that the pain is mainly in the anterior shoulder but can radiate all the way to her wrist. Pain is worsened with reaching, and she is very limited in her ability to reach overhead or behind her back. Cervical motion has no effect on her pain. What are the essential examination elements?

3. The patient has a normal neurologic examination but significant restrictions in both active and passive range of motion of the shoulder in all planes but especially with external rotation and abduction. She has pain with Hawkin's and Neer's maneuvers but a negative empty can test. Her cervical range of motion is full without reproduction of typical pain. Spurling's maneuver is negative. What is your differential? What diagnostic testing, if any, is indicated?

4. X-rays demonstrate mild degenerative changes in the acromio-clavicular joint but otherwise a normal glenohumeral joint and no bony abnormality. How do you counsel the patient about the natural history of her condition?

5. What treatments are available to her?

6. She works as a receptionist in a dental office. She asks whether this condition is work related and if she can make a Workers Compensation claim. How should you respond?

CASE 1: SHOULDER PAIN IN MIDDLE AGE

Answers

1. Key history elements include type of onset (insidious or traumatic), main location of pain (anterior lateral shoulder, superior shoulder, scapular region), exacerbating factors (reaching overhead, behind), alleviating factors, any associated pain sleeping on the shoulder at night time (common symptom of rotator cuff pathology), any symptoms worsened with cervical motion (to assess possible cervical source for pain), and underlying diabetes or thyroid disorders that can predispose the patient to adhesive capsulitis.

2. Essential examination elements include active and passive shoulder range of motion, assessment of upper extremity strength, sensation, reflexes, presence of painful arc (60°–120° shoulder abduction) that is seen in rotator cuff impingement, special shoulder tests (Hawkin's, Neer's, empty can), cervical spine range of motion, palpation, and Spurling's maneuver (Figure 7.1).

3. Differential diagnosis includes rotator cuff impingement/tear, adhesive capsulitis, and glenohumeral osteoarthritis. Tests should include x-rays with the following views—AP, Grashey, and axillary. Ultrasound of the shoulder may show rotator cuff disorders.

4. The patient likely has adhesive capsulitis. Patients with adhesive capsulitis generally present with restrictions in both active *and* passive range of motion, as opposed to rotator cuff disease where active range of motion is restricted but passive range of motion is approximately normal. Glenohumeral osteoarthritis can present with both passive and active range of motion loss but in this case the absence of degenerative changes of the glenohumeral joint on x-rays make osteoarthritis less likely. Discuss that the natural history resolves over 1 to 2 years. Most interventions have not been found to change the natural history.

5. Treatment includes physical therapy focused on improving function, pain control, range of motion, and scapular and rotator cuff strengthening. Oral analgesics for pain should be prescribed, usually nonsteroidals if no contraindications. Intra-articular injections of steroid or hydrodilation with large volumes of normal saline can be beneficial. Manipulation under anesthesia is reserved for refractory cases.

6. Get a thorough history of details of her job. A receptionist generally does not have excessive use of her shoulder to explain this. The patient's condition likely is covered by medical insurance but not Workers Compensation. She can get unpaid time off from work for therapies or doctors' appointments under the Family Medical Leave Act.

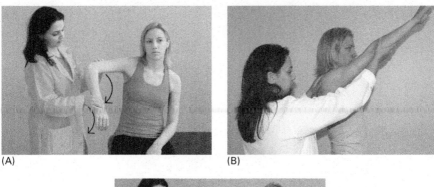

(A)   (B)

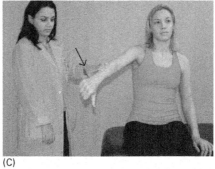

(C)

Figure 7.1   (A) Hawkin's, **(B)** Neer's, and **(C)** empty can tests.

BIBLIOGRAPHY

Andrews J. Frozen shoulder In: Armstrong AD, Hubbard MC, eds. *Essentials of Musculoskeletal Care*. 3rd ed. Rosemont, IL: American Academy of Orthopedic Surgeons; 2005:184-185.

Hsu JE, Anakwenze OA, Warrender WJ, Abboud JA. Current review of adhesive capsulitis. *J Shoulder Elbow Surg.* 2011;20(3):502-514.

Rill BK, Fleckensetin CM, Levy MS, et al. Predictors of outcome after nonoperative and operative treatment of adhesive capsulitis. *Am J Sports Med.* 2011;39(3):567-574.

CASE 2: SHOULDER PAIN—SPORTS RELATED

An 18-year-old male college football player presents to your office with complaints of right shoulder pain and weakness after playing in a game.

Questions

1. What key elements do you want to know from his history?

2. He tells you that he fell backward on his arm and felt that his shoulder "popped out" but was able to later "pop it back in" after a maneuver by the team's athletic trainer. He now has difficulty elevating his arm to comb his hair. What are the essential examination elements?

3. Examination reveals partial weakness of right shoulder abduction and shoulder external rotation and a well-circumscribed area of decreased sensation over the lateral shoulder. He has minimal discomfort with Hawkin's and Neer's maneuvers. Empty can maneuver is negative. Cervical range of motion is normal without pain and Spurling's maneuver is negative. What is your differential diagnosis for his weakness? What diagnostic testing, if any, is indicated and when should it be done?

4. X-ray and MRI of the shoulder demonstrate a Hill-Sach's lesion but normal rotator cuff tendons and labrum. X-ray and MRI of the cervical spine are normal. Axillary motor NCS demonstrate normal distal latency but decreased amplitude. Needle EMG demonstrated the presence of fibrillation potentials in the deltoid and teres minor muscles. Motor unit analysis of these muscles demonstrated decreased motor recruitment. All other muscles tested were normal. What treatments are available to him?

5. Explain his condition to him.

6. He has a big game next week and wants to know when he can return to play. How do you counsel him?

CASE 2: SHOULDER PAIN—SPORTS RELATED

Answers

1. Details of any trauma are key. Did he fall on an outstretched and externally rotated arm (shoulder dislocation)? Direct fall on the shoulder (AC joint injury)? Depression of shoulder while neck laterally rotated (stinger/burner)? Was there presence of neck pain, numbness/tingling, or weakness?

2. Essential examination elements include active and passive shoulder range of motion, upper extremity strength, sensation, reflexes, special shoulder tests (Hawkin's, Neer's, empty can), cervical spine range of motion, palpation, and Spurling's maneuver.

3. Differential diagnosis includes C5-C6 radiculopathy, brachial plexopathy (upper trunk), and shoulder dislocation with axillary nerve injury. Diagnostic testing includes electrodiagnostic studies to evaluate for peripheral nerve injury versus brachial plexopathy versus radiculopathy; x-rays of the shoulder and cervical spine to evaluate for fracture, MRI of the shoulder to evaluate for rotator cuff tear (supraspinatus) and signs of anterior shoulder dislocation (Hill Sachs lesion [Figure 7.2], Bankart lesion), and cervical spine to evaluate for cervical nerve root impingement.

4. Treatments include sling for comfort for a few days; physical therapy to strengthen shoulder abductors, dynamic shoulder stabilizers (rotator cuff), and scapular stabilizers; and oral analgesics.

5. You need to explain his injury in lay terms. He has injured his axillary nerve. He has decreased but good recruitment on electrodiagnostic studies that is suggestive of a good prognosis for recovery. This means that the nerve is still working, but has mild damage. It should recover over the next month or two.

6. He is unlikely to play in the game next week. He will need full pain-free shoulder range of motion and strength before advancing to sport-specific drills and then contact practice. This can take weeks.

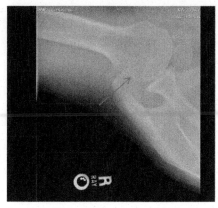 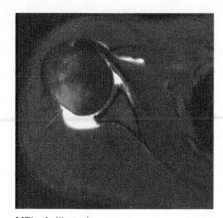

X-ray—Axillary   MRI—Axillary view

Figure 7.2 Hill Sach's lesion.

BIBLIOGRAPHY

Kibler WB, Murrell AC. Shoulder pain. In: Brukner P, Khan K, eds. *Brukner & Khan's Clinical Sports Medicine*. 4th ed. North Ryde, Australia: McGraw-Hill; 2012:242-289.

Robinson CM, Shur N, Sharpe T, et al. Injuries associated with traumatic anterior glenohumeral dislocations. *J Bone Joint Surg Am*. 2012;94(1):18-26.

A 48-year-old, right-hand dominant electrician with a 5-month history of persistent pain in his right elbow presents to your office. The pain was of insidious onset with no precipitating injury or trauma. He is having difficulty performing his job duties, including gripping and using tools.

Questions

1. What key elements do you want to know from his history?

2. He tells you the pain is mostly over the lateral aspect of his right elbow but does radiate along the lateral forearm. It had insidious onset. He has no pain in the neck, arm, or beyond the wrist. He is an electrician. What are the essential examination elements?

3. The patient has a normal neurologic examination. There is point tenderness over the lateral epicondyle, especially a few millimeters distal to the tip of the lateral epicondyle. Resisted wrist extension with elbow extended and forearm pronated, resisted extension of the long finger, and maximal wrist flexion all increase pain at the lateral epicondyle. What is your differential diagnosis? What diagnostic testing is indicated?

4. X-rays (AP/lateral of elbow) were normal. A point-of-care limited diagnostic musculoskeletal ultrasound of the lateral elbow revealed hypoechoic swelling of the common extensor tendon (>4.2 mm) without associated tear. What treatments are available to him?

5. He works as an electrician, but is finding it difficult to perform his job duties. What advice would you give him regarding activity modification and return to activity?

6. Explain his diagnosis, treatment, and prognosis to him in lay terms.

CASE 3: ELBOW PAIN

Answers

1. Key elements of the history include the location of the pain (diffuse pain over the lateral epicondyle and proximal forearm), type of onset (insidious versus traumatic, recent changes in training, technique, duties, or equipment used in sport or work), exacerbating factors (repetitive wrist extension, gripping), alleviating factors, severity of the pain, associated symptoms (absence of neck, upper thoracic, or shoulder pain; absence of sensory symptoms), and activity history (recent change in activities).

2. Essential examination elements include observation, active and passive elbow (flexion/extension, supination/pronation) and wrist (flexion/extension) range of motion, resisted movements including wrist extension with the elbow extended and forearm pronated (Cozen test), grip test and resisted extension of the third metacarpophalangeal joint, palpation (lateral epicondyle, extensor muscles), and neurologic examination of the cervical spine (upper extremity strength, reflex, sensation testing).

3. The most likely diagnosis is lateral epicondylitis. The differential diagnosis includes referred pain from the cervical and upper thoracic spine, synovitis of the radiohumeral joint, radiohumeral bursitis, posterior interosseous nerve entrapment (radial tunnel syndrome), and osteochondritis dissecans. Diagnostic tests are usually not needed but may be ordered to rule out other causes. These may include plain radiographs of elbow (AP, lateral), diagnostic musculoskeletal ultrasound, and MRI imaging of the elbow.

4. Treatments include correcting predisposing factors, physical therapy (eccentric exercise program), therapeutic ultrasound, friction massage, counterforce bracing, wrist immobilization splints, and corticosteroid injection. There is a growing, though still controversial, body of evidence that platelet-rich plasma injections may help in refractory cases. Surgery is reserved for cases that fail conservative management.

5. It is important to correct predisposing factors. These may include equipment use such as modifying the type of screwdriver or other tool, changing grip size, and using proper mechanics. Return to work activities involving repetitive wrist extension and gripping should be gradual and take place over 3 to 6 weeks (varies depending on severity).

6. Describe lateral epicondylitis in lay terms as irritated tendon. Explain each treatment in eighth grade language. Most people's symptoms go away in several weeks.

BIBLIOGRAPHY

Ihm J, Mautner K, Blazuk J, Singh JR. Point/counterpoint. Platelet-rich plasma versus an eccentric exercise program for recalcitrant lateral elbow tendinopathy. *PM R.* 2015;7(6):654-661.

Scott A, Bell S, Vicenzino B. Elbow and arm pain. In: Brukner P, Khan K, eds. *Brukner & Khan's Clinical Sports Medicine.* 4th ed. North Ryde, Australia: McGraw-Hill Education; 2012:390-401.

Woodley BL, Newsham-West RJ, Baxter GD. Chronic tendinopathy: effectiveness of eccentric exercise. *Br J Sports Med.* 2007;41(4):188-198; discussion 199. doi:10.1136/bjsm.2006.

CASE 4: ANKLE SPRAIN

A 24-year-old woman presents to your office one day after injuring her right ankle while playing basketball. She was dribbling up court when the defender attempted to steal the ball from her and in the process stepped forcibly on her anterior ankle. She is having difficulty ambulating without assistance due to pain.

Questions

1. What key elements do you want to know from the history?

2. She is having pain diffusely over the anterior ankle and medial ankle. There is associated swelling. She is unable to weight-bear without significant pain and is using crutches she borrowed from a friend. What are the essential examination elements?

3. The patient has a normal neurologic examination. There is tenderness to palpation over the anterior inferior tibiofibular ligament (AITFL) and posterior aspect of the medial malleolus; there is no tenderness over the proximal fibula; squeeze test is positive; and the external rotation test is positive. What is your differential diagnosis?

4. What diagnostic tests are indicated?

5. Radiographs of the entire tibia and fibula, AP, lateral, and mortise views of the ankle are all negative. What treatment do you recommend?

6. What is the expected return to play timeline?

7. Explain to the patient her condition and prognosis.

CASE 4: ANKLE SPRAIN

Answers

1. Key elements of the history include mechanism of injury (inversion, eversion, compression), onset of pain (ability to weight-bear immediately versus unable to weight-bear), location of pain and swelling (indicates which ligament is involved), degree of swelling and bruising, degree of disability, previous history of ankle injury, and use of protective tape or bracing.

2. Essential examination elements include observation (standing, supine), testing active and passive movements (plantarflexion/dorsiflexion, inversion/eversion), resisted movements (especially eversion in chronic injuries, assessing ankle evertor weakness), functional tests (lunge test, hopping), palpation (distal and proximal fibula, posterior edge/tip of medial and lateral malleolus, base of the fifth metatarsal, anteroinferior tibiofibular ligament, navicular, midfoot zone), and special tests (anterior drawer, talar tilt).

3. The differential diagnosis includes syndesmotic sprain (anteroinferior tibiofibular ligament injury), medial (deltoid) ligament sprain, medial malleolus fracture, tibialis posterior tendon injury, osteochondral lesion, or fracture of the talar dome.

4. Diagnostic testing is warranted given the concern for syndesmotic injury, tenderness to palpation along the posterior aspect of the medial malleolus, and the inability to weight-bear. She satisfies criteria for plain film imaging based on the Ottawa Ankle Rules, which state x-rays are warranted in the setting of malleolar zone pain and tenderness at the posterior edge or tip of the lateral or medial malleolus. X-rays of the ankle include AP, lateral, and mortise views. Include x-rays of the tibia and fibula if there is concern for syndesmotic injury to rule out Maisonneuve fracture. Rarely, an MRI is warranted to evaluate the extent of AITFL injury.

5. If there is no widening of the distal tibiofibular joint, conservative management is appropriate with relative rest and gradual progression to range of motion exercises, strengthening, and proprioceptive retraining. Syndesmotic injuries generally take longer to rehabilitate than lateral ankle sprains.

6. When functional exercises can be performed without pain during or after exercise then progression to return to sport is appropriate. This often is approximately 10 weeks or longer for severe sprains.

7. Using lay terms, explain that she has a moderately severe medial ankle sprain (likely grade 3 of 4). Describe RICE (rest, ice, compression, elevation) and then exercise.

BIBLIOGRAPHY

Bruckner P, Khan K, Hutchison M, et al. Leg pain. In: Bahr R, Blair S, Cook J, et al., eds. *Bruckner & Khan's Clinical Sports Medicine*. 4th ed. Sydney, Australia: McGraw-Hill; 2012:735-760.

Kirschner J. Ankle sprain. *Knowledge NOW*. 2016. Available at: http://me.aapmr.org/kn/article.html?id=111.

Verhagen E, Karlsson J. Acute ankle injuries. In: Brukner P, Khan K, eds. *Brukner & Khan's Clinical Sports Medicine*. 4th ed. North Ryde, Australia: McGraw-Hill Education; 2012:806-827.

CASE 5: KNEE PAIN IN OLDER PATIENT

Mr. James is a 67-year-old gentleman who presents with chronic bilateral knee pain. The pain started 5 years ago and is progressive. Currently, the pain is worse with movement and improved with rest. He does admit the right knee is swollen during the last 3 months.

Questions

1. What information would you like to obtain on history and physical examination?

2. What is your next step? Should a procedure be performed? Imaging (if so, what modality and what views)?

3. Mr. James returns after 2 weeks and complains that pain and decreased range of motion limit his participation in therapy (or home exercise). He asks if an MRI is reasonable or if there is anything else you can do for the pain. X-rays show moderate osteoarthritis and a right knee effusion. What is the next step in management?

4. Aspiration was performed in the right knee and 30 cc of clear yellow fluid was obtained. Should this fluid be sent for analysis?

5. Mr. James returns in 6 weeks as scheduled. He is feeling 60% better. A physician friend of his ordered an MRI of his right knee and he provides you with the study. The images and report indicate a right medial meniscal tear. He asks for the name of an orthopedic surgeon for potential knee arthroscopy. How would you respond?

6. Describe how you might initiate a quality improvement project to limit unnecessary ordering of MRIs in patients with knee pain in your practice.

CASE 5: KNEE PAIN IN OLDER PATIENT

Answers

1. Did the patient have any trauma, fever, chills, or locking or catching of the knee on flexion and extension? Examinations should include strength, range of motion, inspection, palpation, and special tests for meniscal pathology. There is a 2+ effusion to the right knee and a trace effusion on the left. McMurray's test is positive bilaterally. Strength is 5/5. Some redness surrounds the right knee.

2. Weight-bearing x-rays should be ordered (PA in 30° of flexion and lateral). An MRI is not indicated. A course of physical therapy or home exercise would be reasonable with the provision of an NSAID or Tylenol. Opiate pain medications would be less than ideal at this point. Draining the right knee with a corticosteroid injection in the right knee and/or the left knee is reasonable; however, x-rays should be obtained first.

3. Arthrocentesis followed by a corticosteroid injection into the right and, potentially, the left knee is very reasonable at this point.

4. Given the history and physical (no symptoms or signs of infection or inflammatory disease), the fluid can be discarded.

5. It should be explained to Mr. James that there is no evidence that arthroscopic surgery is helpful for an atraumatic meniscal tear. There is a very high rate of asymptomatic tears and the tear apparent on MRI may not be causing his pain. After this explanation, the name of a surgeon or orthopedic practice should, of course, be provided at the patient's request for a second opinion.

6. Unfortunately, there are no published guidelines of criteria for knee MRI. However, you could as a first step do a retrospective chart review of how often the MRI affected management and look at different subgroups—acute injuries versus chronic arthritic pain. Based on these data, reach a consensus among your colleagues of reasonable criteria. Distribute these not only to physicians but patients as well. Then prospectively monitor the number of MRIs ordered, how many were normal, and how many provided information irrelevant to the treatment plan.

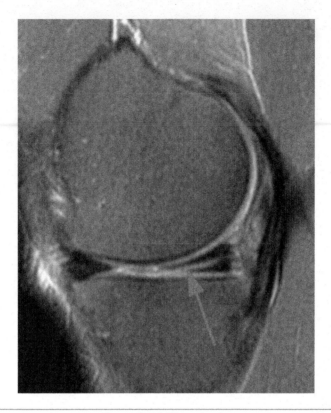

Figure 7.3 MRI meniscal tear.

BIBLIOGRAPHY

Bhattacharyya T, Gale D, Dewire P, et al. The clinical importance of meniscal tears demonstrated by magnetic resonance imaging in osteoarthritis of the knee. *J Bone Joint Surg Am.* 2003;85-A:4-9.

Hepper CT, Halvorson JJ, Duncan ST, et al. The efficacy and duration of injection for knee osteoarthritis. *Sport Med.* 2009;17(10):638-646.

Krych AJ, Johnson NR, Mohan R, et al. Partial meniscectomy provides no benefit for symptomatic degenerative medial meniscus posterior root tears. *Knee Surg Sports Traumatol Arthrosc.* February 9, 2017. doi:10.1007/s00167-017-4454 -5. [Epub ahead of print]

Uthman I, Raynauld J-P, Haraoui B. Intra-articular therapy in osteoarthritis. *Postgrad Med J.* 2003;79(934):449-453.

CASE 6: SHOULDER PAIN IN OLDER PATIENT

A 62-year-old man who is an avid golfer comes to your office with a chief complaint of right shoulder pain and weakness for 4 weeks.

Questions

1. What information is important to obtain on history?

2. There was no acute trauma. The pain came on gradually and is located in the anterior aspect of the right shoulder. No radiation of pain into the right hand is described. Pain is worse with overhead activities. What physical examination will you perform?

3. He lacks full active range of motion on the right in abduction. Strength in external rotation on the right is 2+/5. Impingement signs are positive as is the drop arm test. There is moderate scapular dyskinesis. What is your differential diagnosis and next step?

4. The patient returns in 1 week and is still complaining of pain. His primary physician ordered an MRI at his request, and it shows a partial tear of the right supraspinatus. How does this change your management?

5. Discuss this development with the patient.

6. What are return-to-play guidelines for the patient to resume his golf game?

CASE 6: SHOULDER PAIN IN OLDER PATIENT

Answers

1. History should include recent trauma, prior injury, prior and current function, character and location of pain, exacerbating and remitting factors, and radiation of pain.

2. Examination should include strength testing, sensory examination, reflexes, shoulder and neck active and passive range of motion, and assessment of scapular motion.

3. Differential diagnosis includes rotator cuff tear, impingement syndrome, acromioclavicular joint arthritis, and glenohumeral joint arthritis. Next steps may include ultrasound or MRI and physical therapy for rotator cuff strengthening, as well as scapular stabilization.

4. Management does not change. There is no evidence to support operative management of atraumatic rotator cuff tears.

5. Counsel the patient that he can avoid the difficulties of surgery through a course of physical therapy and continued home exercise.

6. When functional exercises can be performed without pain during or after exercise then progression to return to sport is appropriate.

BIBLIOGRAPHY

Kibler WB, Murrell AC. Shoulder pain. In Brukner P, Khan K, eds. *Brukner & Khan's Clinical Sports Medicine*. 4th ed. North Ryde, Australia: McGraw-Hill; 2012: 242-289.

Tashjian RZ. Epidemiology, natural history, and indications for treatment of rotator cuff tears. *Clin Sports Med.* 2012;31(4):589-604.

Tempelhof S, Rupp S, Seil R. Age-related prevalence of rotator cuff tears in asymptomatic shoulders. *J Shoulder Elbow Surg.* 1999;8(4):296-299.

CASE 7: CHRONIC ANKLE PAIN IN A RUNNER

A 34-year-old woman is an avid runner and presents with 2 months of right ankle pain. The pain came on gradually but yesterday she felt extreme pain during her run and was unable to continue.

Questions

1. What are important elements of the history and physical?

2. Pain is aching and sharp and located at the mid-portion of the Achilles tendon. Pain is worse with movement and improved with rest. Thompson's test is negative. There is swelling and significant pain to the mid-portion of the right Achilles tendon. What is your differential diagnosis?

3. What is your next step? Is any imaging required?

4. What treatment would you recommend?

5. Explain her condition and treatment plan in lay terms.

6. She returns 2 weeks later, and pain has improved to the point where she can run again. She went to one session of physical therapy but has not been back. She has a high co-pay for physical therapy. She asks if physical therapy is indeed indicated in this case.

CASE 7: CHRONIC ANKLE PAIN IN A RUNNER

Answers

1. Important elements of the history include the location and character of the pain, the timing of the pain with running, any exacerbating activities, and any treatments or workup to date. The ankle should be inspected for erythema, instability, and tenderness. The medial and lateral ligaments should be examined as well as the Achilles tendon. For the latter, the Thompson test may be performed.

2. Differential diagnosis includes Achilles tendinosis, Achilles tendon tear, and calf strain.

3. No imaging is required. No further diagnostic testing is warranted.

4. RICE (rest, ice, compression, elevation) should be attempted to ease this acute flare. This should be followed by re-evaluation and potential exercise therapy for the more chronic element of the tendinosis. Eccentric calf strengthening is the cornerstone of treatment for Achilles tendinosis. Other options that can be tried concurrently include active release techniques.

5. Use eighth grade-level language, minimizing words with more than three syllables. Exercises can be demonstrated.

6. She is doing well, and if she understands her home exercises and can demonstrate proper technique to you, there is no need for further physical therapy, which can be quite expensive. She should gradually return to running, monitoring herself closely for exacerbations.

BIBLIOGRAPHY

Smith CC, Syrkin G. Achilles tendinopathy. *Knowledge NOW.* 2013. Available at: http://me.aapmr.org/kn/article.html?id=108.

Van Dijk CN. Mid-portion Achilles tendinopathy: why painful? An evidence-based philosophy. *Knee Surg Sports Traumatol Arthrosc.* 2011;19(8):1367-1375.

Wiegerinck JI, Kerkhoffs GM, van Sterkenburg MN, et al. Treatment for insertional Achilles tendinopathy: a systematic review. *Knee Surg Sports Traumatol Arthrosc.* 2013;21:1345-1355

CASE 8: ACUTE KNEE PAIN IN ADOLESCENT ATHLETE

A 16-year-old high school football player comes to your office after injuring his right knee the day before. He complains of pain and swelling and an inability to flex his knee.

Questions

1. What are important elements of the history and physical?

2. The knee was injured without contact with another player while running forward and attempting to stop and change directions. Swelling occurred immediately, and he is unable to bear weight. There is not bony tenderness, but there is significant tenderness to the knee. Lachman's test is negative. There is a 2+ effusion. What is your next step in the workup?

3. What are immediate interventions to assist the patient?

4. The MRI shows a complete ACL tear. What is your next step in management?

5. The patient asks, "Will I be able to play in 2 weeks? It's the championship game. What if I don't get the surgery, can I play then?"

6. He is very upset by your answer. How would you explain this to him?

CASE 8: ACUTE KNEE PAIN IN ADOLESCENT ATHLETE

Answers

1. Important elements include mechanism of injury, pain level, and pain with weight-bearing. Lachman's test can be performed but will likely be negative at this point in the patient's care.

2. An x-ray should be immediately obtained followed by a right knee MRI without contrast.

3. Advise the patient regarding RICE. Provide a knee immobilizer and crutches. Crutch training would be ideal and is often available at a local physical therapy facility.

4. Referral for orthopedic evaluation is the next step.

5. The patient should be counseled that surgery is very often the next step in this situation given his age and activity level. Unfortunately, he would be unable to play for several weeks with or without surgery.

6. You should express empathy for his situation, but remind him that at his age, he potentially has a long athletic career ahead of him, and he should not risk permanent damage to his knee.

BIBLIOGRAPHY

Laskowsky E. ACL injury and rehabilitation. *Knowledge NOW.* 2016. Available at: http://me.aapmr.org/kn/article.html ?id=109.

Micheo WM, Hernandez L, Seda C. Evaluation, management, rehabilitation, and prevention of anterior cruciate ligament injury: current concepts. *Phys Med Rehabil.* 2010;2:935-944.

CASE 9: HIP PAIN IN AN ATHLETE

A healthy 32-year-old female tennis player presents to your sports medicine clinic with the chief complaint of right hip pain.

Questions

1. What questions would you ask to further determine the cause of the pain?

2. You learn that her pain started 3 weeks ago while she was playing tennis. She was shuffling laterally to her right side to hit a ball when she noticed the pain. The pain is located in the groin and lateral hip. There is some pain in the anterior thigh, but it is primarily located in the groin. The pain is a constant dull ache with intermittent sharp, stabbing pains with activity. It has worsened with time as she has continued to play tennis and work out. The pain is worsened with activity such as walking, pivoting/turning, or playing tennis and improved with rest but there is also discomfort with prolonged sitting. She denies numbness, tingling, and weakness. No popping or locking of the hip occurs but she does feel unstable at times. She has no history of stress fractures or bone density problems. She has no dietary restrictions. Age of menarche 13, normal menses. What would you include on physical exam?

3. On physical exam, she has an antalgic gait. There is tenderness to palpation of the anterior hip and minimal tenderness over the lateral hip. She has normal strength and neurologic exam. Her lumbar spine and knee range of motion are normal and pain-free. Passive hip range of motion on the left is normal and pain-free. On the right, she has pain with hip flexion and internal rotation and restricted internal rotation range. She has positive FADIR (flexion, adduction, internal rotation) and hip scour. Stinchfield (resisted straight leg raise) is positive. Patrick's/FABER (flexion, abduction, and external rotation) is negative and provides some relief of pain. Heel strike and fulcrum test are negative. Hop test is painful on the right. She demonstrates weakness of hip abductors with single-leg squat. What is the differential diagnosis? What diagnostic testing is indicated?

4. X-rays of the right hip demonstrate small cam deformity with minimal degenerative changes. Diagnostic hip injection is positive in that her pain resolves. MR arthrogram demonstrates a small superior acetabular labral tear and minimal degenerative changes of the right hip. What treatment would you recommend?

5. The patient is concerned that physical therapy is just a waste of time and money and asks why you're not just referring her to the surgeon first. How would you counsel her?

6. How might the approach differ if she were a professional athlete versus a recreational player?

CASE 9: HIP PAIN IN AN ATHLETE

Answers

1. When did the pain start? Was there a specific injury/mechanism? Where is the pain located (groin pain vs. trochanteric)? Does the pain radiate? What is the severity of the pain? What is the quality of the pain? What has been the progression? What aggravates the pain? What alleviates the pain? What is her current activity level? Prior hip injuries? Review of systems includes numbness/tingling, weakness, popping/locking/instability (mechanical symptoms). What treatments has she tried? History of stress fractures, bone density problems, dietary restrictions, menstrual history? Past medical history? Social history including alcohol use (risk factor for AVN)?

2. Physical exam includes general appearance, gait, and muscle strength; the neurologic exam includes reflexes and sensation in the lower extremities; exam of the lumbar spine, hip, knee range of motion, palpation of lumbar spine and hip girdle; special tests include FABER/Patrick's, FADIR, hip scour, and heel strike/hop/fulcrum (stress fracture tests). Can also include functional evaluation of hip abductor strength through single-leg stance and single-leg squat.

3. Differential diagnosis includes hip impingement, hip osteoarthritis, labral tear, femoral stress fracture, avascular necrosis, lumbar radiculitis, and femoral neuropathy. Primary hip joint pathology is the most likely pain generator given the location of her pain and reproduction with FADIR and hip scour maneuvers. Tests include hip x-ray (including AP and lateral views), diagnostic hip injection with lidocaine ± steroid (if x-rays are negative, that can confirm intra-articular source of pain), and MR arthrogram of the hip (MRI to evaluate for stress fracture and arthrogram to evaluate for labral tear).

4. Treatment options include analgesic medications as needed for pain (acetaminophen, NSAIDs); activity modification to avoid aggravating activities; physical therapy to address possible biomechanical deficits and weakness, and opportunities to teach appropriate movements; intra-articular steroid injection can be utilized if other treatments fail; ultimately, the patient can be referred to an orthopedic surgeon if conservative measures fail to relieve pain and/or allow return to activity.

5. First you want to reassure the patient that you understand her concerns and that there is no harm done in waiting for surgery. Discuss that physical therapy is the appropriate first-line treatment and can provide good resolution of symptoms and allow return to sport and desired activities without surgery, which carries higher risks and also does not guarantee a successful outcome. Physical therapy can address the biomechanical issues and weaknesses that contributed to injury and will be helpful in the long run even if she does proceed to surgery—it can be thought of as "pre-habilitation."

6. The overall approach should be the same. However, she may have resources for more frequent and intensive physical therapy. As her livelihood is at stake, earlier referral to surgery may be warranted.

BIBLIOGRAPHY

Bruckner P, Khan K, Kemp J, et al. Hip-related pain. In: Bahr R, Blair S, Cook J, et al., eds. *Brukner & Khan's Clinical Sports Medicine.* 4th ed. Sydney, Australia: McGraw-Hill; 2012:510-544.
Groh MM, Herrera J. A comprehensive review of hip labral tears. *Curr Rev Musculoskeletal Med.* 2009;2(2):105-117.
Prather H, Colorado B, Hunt D. Managing hip pain in the athlete. *Phys Med Rehabil Clin N Am.* 2014;25:789-812.

CASE 10: LEG PAIN IN AN ADOLESCENT RUNNER

A healthy 15-year-old male high school cross country athlete presents to your sports medicine clinic with the chief complaint of left leg pain.

Questions

1. What questions would you ask to further determine the cause of the pain?

2. The pain is located in the anterior medial shin. His pain started 3 weeks ago as he started increasing the distances he was running in cross-country practices with his school team. He had been training over the summer but significantly increased his mileage when starting practices with school. He has been running on paved surfaces recently but worked out on the track during the summer. Pain is absent at rest. With activity, pain is located anteriorly in the right shin and is rated 8/10. Initially, pain would subside as he continued running, but now it persists. He has had to stop running due to the pain. The pain has improved somewhat since he stopped running in the last few days. Pain worsens with walking and running and is improved with rest. He denies numbness, tingling, weakness, and lower extremity swelling. What would you do on your physical exam?

3. On exam, he has symmetric 2+ dorsalis pedis and posterior tibial pulses. Strength and sensation are normal in the lower extremities. He has increased pronation with ambulation. There is diffuse tenderness to palpation along the middle third of the posteromedial tibial border. He has reduced dorsiflexion range of motion with the knee flexed. He has pain reproduction with the tuning fork test. What is your differential diagnosis? What would you do to test your differential and determine the diagnosis?

4. X-ray of the leg is negative. MRI demonstrates periosteal edema on T2-weighted images along the middle third of the posteromedial tibial border. You diagnose medial tibial stress syndrome. What would you recommend next?

5. He has an important cross country meet in a week and wants to compete. How do you counsel him and his parents regarding this?

6. His coach calls you after the visit and wants to know why you won't let him run in the meet. How should you respond?

CASE 10: LEG PAIN IN AN ADOLESCENT RUNNER

Answers

1. Where is the pain located? What is the severity of the pain? What is the quality of the pain? When did the pain start? Were there any changes in training or exercise at that time? What has been the progression? What aggravates the pain? What alleviates the pain? Is there pain with weight-bearing or walking? What is his current activity level? How does the pain change with activity? Any prior leg injuries? Review of systems includes weakness, numbness/tingling, cramping, and swelling.

2. Physical exam includes neurologic exam of reflexes and strength. Cardiovascular exam of distal pulses is performed. Include inspection of lower extremity alignment, foot structure, and ankle/foot alignment with ambulation. Palpate along the medial tibial border to determine if a focal or more diffuse area of pain. Evaluate range of motion of the ankle and foot including with knee flexed and extended to assess for both gastrocnemius and soleus tightness. Perform a tuning fork test. Should also include an evaluation of hip and knee range of motion.

3. Differential diagnosis includes MTSS (shin splints), tibial stress fracture, chronic exertional compartment syndrome, muscle strain, vascular compression (usually popliteal), metabolic bone disease, bony tumor (osteosarcoma, osteoid osteoma), and lumbar radicular pain. Tests include x-rays to evaluate for obvious stress fracture but will often be negative even in the setting of fracture. Bone scans are not as specific as MRI, which is a test of choice as it can differentiate MTSS and stress fracture and help grade stress fractures, which can direct treatment and provide prognostic information. Other tools in evaluation of exertional leg pain include compartment pressure testing (pre- and postexertion), ABI, MR angiogram, and EMG/NCS. CT is not indicated and increases radiation in a young patient.

4. Treatment includes rest from aggravating activities and treating the underlying pathology. Ice and analgesics (acetaminophen, NSAIDs) can be used. The patient should be allowed to cross-train with pain-free activities such as swimming or cycling to maintain cardiovascular fitness. Immobilization and protected weight-bearing in a knee-high walking boot or pneumatic stirrup leg brace may be required. For excessive pronation, appropriate footwear and orthotics should be recommended. A course of physical therapy to address stretching and strengthening is recommended. When pain free, he can pursue a gradual return to sport.

5. It is important to empathize with him but to advise him of the risks involved if he were to continue to run. There is the possibility that if he continues to run he could develop a stress fracture. That would then be more difficult to manage, potentially requiring a period of nonweight bearing and strict avoidance of activity. There is even the possibility that it would require surgery if he had a higher risk anterior tibial fracture. The appropriate treatment is rest and addressing necessary biomechanical issues to prevent recurrence.

He should then have a quicker and more successful return to sport with lower likelihood of future injuries.

6. It is inappropriate for you to discuss the case with the coach without the patient's and the parent's consent due to privacy laws (HIPAA).

BIBLIOGRAPHY

Bruckner P, Khan K, Hutchison M, et al. Leg pain. In: Bahr R, Blair S, Cook J, et al., eds. *Bruckner & Khan's Clinical Sports Medicine*. 4th ed. Sydney, Australia: McGraw-Hill; 2012:735-760.

Malbrough TJ, Metzler JP. Lower leg injuries and conditions. In Harrast A, Finoff JT, eds. *Sports Medicine Study Guide*, 2nd Ed. New York, NY.; Demos Medical, 2016:315-321.

Rajasekaran S, Finnoff JT. Exertional leg pain. *Phys Med Rehabil Clin N Am*. 2016;27:91-119.

8 Neuromuscular Impairments and Electrodiagnosis

Tae Chung

A 55-year-old man comes to a neuromuscular clinic complaining of numbness and burning sensation in both feet. The symptom started about 2 years ago, and he has no other known past medical history.

Questions

1. What questions would you ask before planning for further diagnostic workup?

2. You learn that his symptoms started gradually about 2 years ago in the bottom of his feet, and slowly progressed to the mid-shin level. It started with severe burning, followed by numbness, and he also feels some weakness in the ankles. The symptoms progressed symmetrically. More recently, he started having some urinary retention and severe constipation. He became a vegan at age 50 to improve his health. He is having trouble in his work as a real estate agent due to limited walking tolerance. His wife says he has become forgetful and clumsy in the past few months. What physical exam findings are important?

3. His exam shows normal strength, except for 4/5 in the dorsiflexion and plantarflexion of both ankles. Sensory deficits are in a length-dependent pattern for all sensory modalities. Proprioception is poor in both great toes. Vibration sense is absent below the knees. Deep tendon reflexes are absent in both ankles, but 3+ in the knees with positive cross-adductor responses bilaterally. He was able to recall one object out of three in a short-term memory test, but his long-term memory is intact. What's in the differential? What diagnostic tests are indicated?

4. His nerve conduction study shows absent sural sensory response, low CMAP amplitudes of bilateral peroneal at extensor digiti brevis (EDB), and bilateral tibial nerves, whereas the motor response of bilateral peroneal at tibialis anterior are normal. EMG shows mild spontaneous activities and several large units with a neurogenic recruitment pattern, only in the tibialis anterior and gastrocnemius muscles, but other muscles are normal. His labs show borderline low serum vitamin B_{12} level but very high serum MMA and high serum homocysteine levels. MRI of the brain and spinal cord is normal. What is the diagnosis, and what treatment would you recommend?

5. At the end of the visit, he reveals that he has been a strict vegan for several years since his brother died of a massive stroke, and he wants to have your opinions on his diet. What advice would you provide to him?

6. If he were a vegan for religious reasons, how might you approach the conversation differently?

CASE 1: POLYNEUROPATHY

Answers

1. Questions should involve the time course/progression of symptoms; distribution of sensory deficits; distribution of motor deficits; how the symptoms limit his daily functions; possibility of exposure to any neurotoxin (e.g., chemotherapeutic agents, vocational exposure, unusual diet, or gastric surgery); and history of diabetes. You also need a complete review of systems.

2. Important physical exam findings include deep tendon reflexes; manual muscle testing; sensory exam with light touch, pinprick, and vibration/position; and brief memory test.

3. Tests indicated include EMG/NCS; CBC; vitamin B_1, B_6, and B_{12} levels; HbA1c (or blood sugar level); MRI of spine; and MRI of brain. Differential diagnosis includes polyneuropathy, myelopathy, subacute combined degeneration, entrapment neuropathy, neuroma, complex regional pain syndrome (CRPS), and multilevel lumbosacral radiculopathy.

4. EMG/NCS shows a length-dependent sensorimotor polyneuropathy; he has a subacute combined degeneration from vitamin B_{12} deficiency, given high MMA and homocysteine level (when serum vitamin B_{12} is borderline low, MMA and homocysteine levels are more sensitive). Treatment includes intramuscular vitamin B_{12} injection for 1 month, followed by oral vitamin B_{12} supplement; physical therapy for strengthening and balance training; and orthotic evaluation.

5. He has subacute combined degeneration from B_{12} deficiency. His vitamin B_{12} neuropathy is likely due to his veganism, given the timeline. The advice to this patient should include (a) risks of extreme diet habits; (b) possible referral to nutritionist; (c) importance of exercise, in addition to diet, for cardiovascular health; (d) communicating with his primary physician regarding his cardiovascular risks and the family history; and (e) dietary recommendations for B_{12}-rich foods.

6. If his veganism was due to religious or moral considerations, you should be nonjudgmental about his diet, and can advise him that supplementation with B_{12} is necessary.

BIBLIOGRAPHY

Amato AA, Dumitru D. Approach to peripheral neuropathy. In: Dumitru D, ed. *Electrodiagnostic Medicine*. 2nd ed. Philadelphia, PA: Hanley & Belfus; 2002:chap 21.

Amato AA, Russell JA. Neuropathies associated with systemic disorder. In: Amato AA, Russell JA, eds. *Neuromuscular Disorder*. New York, NY: McGraw-Hill; 2008:chap 14.

Dombovy ML. Rehabilitation management of neuropathies. In: Dyck PJ, Thomas PK, eds. *Peripheral Neuropathy*. 4th ed. Philadelphia, PA: Elsevier; 2005:2621-2636.

CASE 2: PROGRESSIVE WEAKNESS

A 62-year-old female with progressive muscle weakness is referred to your PM&R clinic. She started having muscle weakness after spine surgery performed about 3 years ago, and now she uses a wheelchair for mobility. She recently developed difficulty swallowing and has a soft voice.

Questions

1. What questions would you ask before planning for further diagnostic workup?

2. She says that she developed right foot drop about 3 years ago, but there was no sensory deficits. She always had very mild back pain, and her neurosurgeon decided to perform spine surgery. However, after the surgery, the weakness worsened and progressed to the right knee, left ankle, and the right hip over the next 1 to 2 years. About a year ago, she developed right wrist drop and some weakness in the left elbow. There has been no sensory deficits or changes in the back pain. What are the important physical findings?

3. Please list the differential diagnosis.

4. You decided to do an electrodiagnostic study. The nerve conduction study shows normal sensory studies in both lower and upper extremities. However, CMAPs of the peroneal, tibial, and right radial motor nerves are all reduced with relatively preserved conduction velocity in an asymmetric pattern. EMG shows 3 to 4+ spontaneous activities and very large units with the neurogenic recruitment pattern in all the muscles from the bulbar, cervical, thoracic, and lumbosacral regions. Fasciculation potentials are frequently seen in multiple muscles. What other diagnostic workups would you recommend, and what is the rationale?

5. All the labs and imaging studies came back negative. What is the presumed diagnosis? What's your approach to the patient for prognostication and what is your treatment plan for her?

6. Explain the disease and prognosis to her in lay terms.

7. At the follow-up visit, she says she recently saw an alternative medicine doctor who says her ALS is related to a subclinical Lyme infection, although she never had any positive Lyme test. She is considering receiving IV doxycycline for 6 months as recommended by the doctor. What advice would you give to her?

CASE 2: PROGRESSIVE WEAKNESS

Answers

1. Questions should involve the time course/progression of symptoms; distribution of sensory symptoms, if any; distribution of motor deficits; how the symptoms limit her daily functions; possible complications from the spine surgery; and progression of back pain. How is this impacting her participation in daily activities?

2. The important physical findings are deep tendon reflexes, upper motor neuron signs (at least two of the following should be done: cross-adduction, Babinski, Hoffman's, jaw jerk), manual muscle testing, sensory exam, inspection of tongue for fasciculation and/or atrophy, and inspection for fasciculation and/or atrophy in limb and trunk muscles.

3. Differential diagnosis includes ALS, multilevel radiculopathy, vasculitic neuropathy, and inclusion body myositis.

4. ALS is a diagnosis of exclusion, and therefore requires a comprehensive workup to rule out other possibilities. Workup: CBC and metabolic panel, toxicity screening (including heavy metal), CPK (and/or aldolase), CSF analysis, MRI of spine, and MRI of brain.

5. The patient meets the El Escorial criteria for the diagnosis of ALS. Treatment plans should include the following: palliative care; riluzole; aggressive pulmonary rehabilitation (should mention CPAP and/or BiPAP +/- CoughAssist); speech evaluation for dysphagia and communication; wheelchair evaluation; physical therapy evaluation for mobility; and occupational therapy evaluation for activities of daily living and adaptive devices.

6. It is important to clearly inform the patient in a sensitive way that ALS is a fatal disease with median life span of less than 5 years. You might start by asking the patient how much she wants to know about the prognosis now. You can emphasize that we can only give average life spans, and that there are some people who are long-term survivors (e.g., Stephen Hawking). You should also initiate a conversation about advance directives. Would she want enteral feedings or home mechanical ventilation?

7. While the association between chronic Lyme and ALS may be controversial, this patient never had a Lyme infection, given the negative Lyme tests. It should be clearly mentioned that the potential risks of IV doxycycline treatment in the absence of Lyme infection will outweigh any potential benefits of the treatment. The consultation should include the following: scientific rationale for alternative treatments; potential risks of alternative treatments; ethical and legal issues involving alternative treatments; and financial issues with alternative care. You should sensitively counsel the patient that many people may offer unproven treatments for her disease, and that she should carefully weigh the evidence for their efficacy and the risks versus benefits.

BIBLIOGRAPHY

Amato AA, Russell JA. Amyotrophic lateral sclerosis. In: Amato AA, Russell JA, eds. *Neuromuscular Disorder*. New York, NY: McGraw-Hill; 2008:chap 4.

de Carvalho M, Dengler R, Eisen A, et al. Electrodiagnostic criteria for diagnosis of ALS. *Clin Neurophys*. 2008;119:497-503.

Howard RS. Respiratory failure because of neuromuscular disease. *Curr Opin Neurol*. October 2016;29(5):592-601.

Kiernan MC, Vucic S. Amyotrophic lateral sclerosis. *Lancet*. March 12, 2011;377(9769):942-955.

CASE 3: PROXIMAL WEAKNESS IN AN ADULT

A 43-year-old female with progressive muscle weakness in her shoulders and hips is referred to your PM&R clinic. She developed muscle weakness about 3 months ago. She also noticed some skin lesions, but denies any pain.

Questions

1. What questions would you ask before planning for further diagnostic workup?

2. She says that she realized one day that she could not comb her hair and stand up from a toilet by herself. She developed the weakness over 3 to 5 days, but didn't have any pain. A few days later, she developed rashes and severe itchiness in the face and knuckles. What are the important physical findings and diagnostic workup? Provide a rationale for each workup as well.

3. A sensory conduction study is normal, but EMG shows small units with early recruitment patterns in proximal muscles (Figure 8.1). A muscle biopsy shows extensive inflammation in the perimysium and endomysium, with perifascicular atrophy (Figure 8.2). What is the diagnosis? What is the next step of workup and treatment?

4. Explain her diagnosis and treatment to her in lay terms.

5. She responded well to the treatments that included high-dose steroids, and now she is walking independently. However, she still has a significant amount of fatigue and some weakness 6 months after the treatment was started. What are the possible reasons and treatments?

6. At the follow-up visit, you notice that her weakness has declined again. She admits that she has been skipping her medications as she has been very busy as a single mother who raises a teenage boy by herself. What would you advise her?

CASE 3: PROXIMAL WEAKNESS IN AN ADULT

Answers

1. Questions involve the time course/progression of symptoms; distribution of sensory symptoms, if any; distribution of muscle weakness; how the symptoms limit her daily functions; any skin lesions; and any joint pain.

2. Physical findings include deep tendon reflexes, manual muscle testing, and sensory exam inspection of skin lesions. Workup includes EMG/NCS; myositis-specific antibodies; CPK (and/or aldolase); MRI of muscle; MRI of spine.

3. Dermatomyositis is the diagnosis. Treatment includes high-dose prednisone (steroid), followed by a secondary agent (i.e., IVIG, methotrexate, Cellcept, Imuran, or rituximab). Physical exercise is also an important treatment modality.

4. You need to use eighth grade-level language and illicit whether she understands what you have explained. Talk about the body's immune system attacking her muscle cells and how medication stops this process.

5. The patient was on high-dose steroids, so the possible reasons for fatigue and continuing weakness include steroid-induced myopathy; side effects from immune medications; Addison's disease; relapse of the dermatomyositis; and disuse atrophy. Depending on the etiology, accepted answers include tapering off steroid; referral to an endocrinologist for evaluation of Addison's disease; reducing the dose of suspected medications; increasing the dose of immune medications for the relapse of dermatomyositis; physical therapy and resistance exercise for disuse atrophy. Psychosocial reasons, such as depression and/or social stress, should be considered, and referral to a psychologist or social worker is also an acceptable answer.

6. Patient education about the importance of immune medications and their potential benefits/risks should be the first step. Ask if her insurance covers the medicine and how high is the co-pay. Is this the issue? If appropriate, referral to social services can be considered. Some pharmaceutical companies offer discounts for patients with financial difficulties.

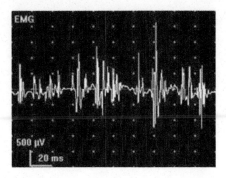

Figure 8.1 EMG small amplitude polyphasic motor unit.

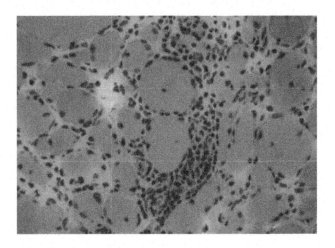

Figure 8.2 Muscle biopsy dermatomyositis.

BIBLIOGRAPHY

Amato AA, Russell JA. Inflammatory myopathies. In: Amato AA, Russell JA, eds. *Neuromuscular Disorder*. New York, NY: McGraw-Hill;2008:chap 30.
Dalakas MC. Inflammatory muscle diseases. *N Engl J Med*. April 30, 2015;372(18):1734-1747.

CASE 4: ENTRAPMENT NEUROPATHY CASE

A right-handed, 33-year-old male is referred to your EMG clinic for evaluation of numbness and tingling in the right hand. He also has occasional neck pain. He is a software engineer who works on a computer all day long.

Questions

1. What questions would you ask before planning for further diagnostic workup?

2. He says the pain started about 3 years ago, but worsened about 6 months ago. He drops things at work. He sometimes wakes up at night due to pain. He is having trouble typing. What are the important physical exam findings and why? What is the most important diagnostic test to order?

3. He has a positive Tinel's and Phalen's test, but negative Spurling's and Hoffman's tests. In the electrodiagnostic study, the right median sensory conduction study shows reduction of the conduction velocity across the wrist, while the left side is normal. CMAP of the right median nerve shows distal latency of 6.0 ms (normal <4.2 ms), and amplitudes are more than 50% reduced in the right side, compared to the left side (5 mV vs. 12 mV). Sensory and motor conduction studies of ulnar and radial nerves are all normal bilaterally. What is the differential diagnosis at this point, and which muscles would you study for EMG? Please provide the rationale for your answers.

4. During the EMG needling of the abductor pollicis brevis muscle, the patient suddenly becomes very anxious due to pain, screaming to stop the EMG study. What would you do in this situation, and what would you do to prevent this from happening in the future?

5. EMG of the abductor digiti minimus and flexor digitorum longus showed no abnormalities. What are the treatment options for this patient?

6. What are appropriate work restrictions or accommodations for this patient?

CASE 4: ENTRAPMENT NEUROPATHY CASE

Answers

1. Questions include time course/progression of symptoms; distribution of sensory symptoms, if any; distribution of motor deficits; how the symptoms limit his daily functions; and the nature of neck pain (radiation, distribution, and frequency).

2. The exam should be focused on common entrapment neuropathy (carpal tunnel and/or cubital tunnel syndrome) and cervical radiculopathy, especially at the C8T1 level. Tests should address deep tendon reflexes; manual muscle testing of median versus ulnar versus radial nerve innervated muscles; sensory exam of median versus ulnar versus radial nerve distribution; inspection of muscle atrophy in the median or ulnar innervated muscles; Tinel's signs at the wrist or elbow. Phalen's sign should also be checked, as it is more sensitive than the Tinel's sign. Any physical exam for cervical radiculopathy should include range of motion, Spurling's signs, and Hoffman's signs. If he has findings consistent with carpal tunnel syndrome, electrodiagnosis would be the best first test to order, as it can also differentiate cervical radiculopathy.

3. He most likely has carpal tunnel syndrome (median neuropathy at the wrist) in the right hand. The severity is at least moderate, given that CMAP is affected. EMG should include at least one median-innervated muscle (such as APB), one ulnar-mediated muscle (such as FDI or ADM), and one median-innervated muscle proximal to carpal tunnel (such as pronator teres or FPL). This can exclude proximal median nerve impingement and cervical radiculopathy. In addition, needle EMG may provide additional data on the severity and prognosis.

4. If the patient has a decision-making capacity, the examiner should respect his wishes and stop the procedure. However, the disadvantage of stopping the procedure should be explained to the patient, and if necessary, the study should be re-attempted. If the patient still refuses the procedure, alternative options should be provided. To minimize the discomfort, the following can be considered: planning to do needling of the most painful muscles at the end, distraction technique by talking to the patient during the procedure, calm environment, and clear prior explanation of the procedure.

5. Splinting is the most reasonable first step. However, given that he has at least moderate severity carpal tunnel syndrome (with motor involvement), surgical consultation for carpal tunnel release should be considered. Other interventions might include ergonomic modification, occupational hand therapy, corticosteroid injection, median nerve gliding exercise, and pain medications (including NSAIDs).

6. Explore whether using voice activated typing would work for him. Adjustments can be made to his keyboard and mouse to make them more ergonomic. He should take rest breaks frequently from typing.

BIBLIOGRAPHY

Amato AA, Russell JA. Cervical and thoracic radiculopathies, brachial plexopathies, and mononeuropathies of the arm. In: Amato AA, Russell JA, eds. *Neuromuscular Disorder.* New York, NY: McGraw-Hill;2008:chap 21.

American Association of Electrodiagnostic Medicine, American Academy of Neurology, and American Academy of Physical Medicine and Rehabilitation. Practice parameter for electrodiagnostic studies in carpal tunnel syndrome: summary statement. *Muscle Nerve.* 2009;25:918-922.

Huisstede BM, Hoogvliet P, Randsdorp MS, et al. Carpal tunnel syndrome. Part I: effectiveness of nonsurgical treatments: a systemic review. *Arch Phys Med Rehab.* 2010;91(7):981-1004.

Huisstede BM, Randsdorp MS, Coert JH, et al. Carpal tunnel syndrome. Part II: effectiveness of surgical treatments: a systemic review. *Arch Phys Med Rehab.* 2010;91(7):1005-1024.

9 Pain and Spinal Impairments

Bryt Christensen and Nathan Neufeld

CASE 1: ABDOMINAL PAIN

A 54-year-old woman presents with epigastric pain, bloating, no nausea and vomiting, worsening pain with eating, and a new diagnosis of pancreatic cancer.

Questions

1. What more do you need to know about her history and physical exam?

2. She has 8/10 epigastric pain with radiation to the mid back. It interferes with sleep, and she has been unable to work. What type of pain is she having? What medications and procedures might be helpful in alleviating her pain?

3. You have opted to start opioid medications for her. How can you mitigate side effects, especially the risk of overdose?

4. Besides opioids and celiac plexus block, what other treatment modalities could be considered?

5. The patient has collected a large bag full of narcotic and pain medications over the last year of her fight with cancer. She wants you to take them because she does not want them around her house. What do you do?

CASE 1: ABDOMINAL PAIN

Answers

1. What is the character of her pain? How severe is it both on an analog scale and how does it interfere with her function?

2. Her pain is visceral in nature. It is likely to respond to opioid medication, but the prescriber needs to be cautious about side effects, including constipation, confusion, diversion to others, and overdose. Pancreatic cancer patients often are helped by a celiac plexus block, which can reduce opioid use.

3. It is very important with narcotic writing to utilize pharmacy databases and communicate clearly with all involved care team members to make sure there is only one narcotic prescribing team. Concomitant prescription of rescue intranasal naloxone has been shown to reduce the risk of overdose death. The patient should keep her medication locked up, as family members are the most likely to divert prescriptions. Constipation should be aggressively managed. The patient and family members should monitor for signs of delirium.

4. Arguably the most important aspect of pain care in cancer patients is that of psychology. All psychological services—psychiatry, psychology, mind-body therapy, counseling, pastoral care, social work, and so on—are of great value to cancer patients. One should screen for depression and anxiety and make appropriate referrals. Complementary and alternative treatments such as acupuncture or massage can be considered as long as the patient understands the limits of evidence supporting their use, and can afford the out of pocket expense.

5. The medications given to the patient by the pharmacy are the patient's property. It is, therefore, not acceptable for the provider or anyone of the care team to take the property from the patient. This can be perceived as stealing, and/ or if medications go missing the care team can be blamed. Even pharmacies are unable to take medications back. Therefore, recommend dissolving the pills in hot water in a bottle and adding coffee grounds in order to dispose of the pills in the trash. It also is not recommended to put pills in the public sewer system.

BIBLIOGRAPHY

Christo PJ, Mazloomdoost D. Interventional pain treatments for cancer pain. *Ann N Y Acad Sci.* 2008;1138(1):299-328.
Drug Enforcement Administration, Department of Justice. Disposal of controlled substances. Final rule. *Fed Regist.* 2014;79(174):53519.
Krajnik M, Zylicz Z. Pain assessment, recognizing clinical patterns and cancer pain syndromes. In Hanna M, Zylicz Z. *Cancer Pain.* London, UK: Springer. 2013;95-108
Gordon DB, Dahl JL, Miaskowski C, et al. American Pain Society recommendations for improving the quality of acute and cancer pain management: American Pain Society Quality of Care Task Force. *Arch Intern Med.* 2005;165(14):1574-1580.

CASE 2: ACUTE SHOULDER PAIN

A 35-year-old man has had right shoulder pain for 1 week, after moving some scrap metal at his home. He is holding his arm and pacing the room.

Questions

1. What are pertinent further questions in the history?

2. He is right handed. Pain is 10/10 in the anterior shoulder, aggravated by any overhead reaching. It hurts when he lies on that right side. The patient has no significant past medical history. He works a sedentary job, and walks for exercise. What physical exam special tests will be most important to make a diagnosis?

3. He has a painful arc from 45 to 120 degrees of abduction, an internal rotation lag, and positive Hawkin's and empty can signs. Drop arm test is negative, as are Spurling's and Adson's signs. Neurologic exam is normal. What is the most likely diagnosis? What diagnostic tests are appropriate at this time?

4. What treatment would you initially order?

5. The patient asks specifically for oxycodone 10 mg and Soma 350 mg. He states that they have worked the best in the past when he had a bout of back pain 2 years ago. How should you react?

6. You advise him to take naproxen 500 mg bid over the counter. He saw an ad on TV for celecoxib and wants a prescription for that because he believes it will work better. How do you proceed?

CASE 2: ACUTE SHOULDER PAIN

Answers

1. Ask which hand is dominant, the character of the pain; alleviating and aggravating factors; if neck, hand, or forearm pain is present; functional limitations; and occupation.

2. Painful arc, internal rotation lag, and Hawkin's sign are the most sensitive and specific tests for rotator cuff tendinosis. Drop arm test can rule out a complete tear. One should also examine the neck to exclude radicular pain.

3. A strong argument could be made against any diagnostic testing this soon after injury, and reserving it for several weeks later if he does not improve with conservative management. However, if there is a more urgent need (e.g., the patient needed to return to work soon and his job required reaching or throwing), either MRI or diagnostic ultrasound would be appropriate (the latter requires an appropriately trained ultrasonographer).

4. The treatment should involve RICE (rest, ice, compression, elevation), external rotation/scapular stabilization, and NSAIDs.

5. Patients can ask for something that they think works best. However, starting with an over-the-counter medicine (such as an NSAID) is always best. Additionally, antispasmodics and muscle relaxants are not first line for acute injury. Narcotics should only be resorted to after other options have failed. We, however, should not assume that the patient is being dishonest and drug seeking.

6. COX-2 inhibitors are no more effective than over-the-counter NSAIDs in equivalent doses, but do have fewer GI side effects. Assuming the patient has not had GI problems, his insurance is unlikely to cover this medication due to its higher cost.

BIBLIOGRAPHY

Curatolo M, Bogduk N. Pharmacologic pain treatment of musculoskeletal disorders: current perspectives and future prospects. *Clin J Pain.* 2001;17(1):25-32.

Dowell D, Haegerich TM, Chou R. CDC guideline for prescribing opioids for chronic pain—United States, 2016. *MMWR Recomm Rep.* 2016;65:1-49.

Kibler WB, Murrell AC. Shoulder pain. In: Brukner P, Khan K, eds. *Clinical Sports Medicine.* 4th ed. North Ryde, Australia: McGraw Hill;2012:242-289.

Van der Windt DA, Koes BW, Boeke AJ, et al. Shoulder disorders in general practice: incidence, patient characteristics, and management. *Ann Rheum Dis.* 1995;54(12):959-964.

CASE 3: LOW BACK PAIN

A 36-year-old woman has had low back pain for 7 years following the birth of her third child. She is finding it more difficult to sit for extended periods of time, especially on the bleachers at her oldest son's basketball games recently. She has seen her primary care physician for this pain before, but he only recommended ibuprofen. Vitals are normal.

1. What key elements do you want to know from her history?

2. She has no "red flags" and no radicular pain. Sitting worsens her pain, while lying down or standing up alleviates it. What physical examination would help determine the origin of the pain?

3. She has no kyphoscoliosis and full range of motion. Straight leg raising is negative. No pain is reported with extension or lateral bending. She has point tenderness over the bilateral SI joints, positive FABER (for buttocks but not groin pain), compression and distraction of the SI joints, and a positive Gaenslen's test. What imaging or diagnostic tests should be ordered?

4. X-ray of the SI joint shows no pathology. HLA-B27 and ESR are normal. What initial therapy would help her "low back pain"? If that is unsuccessful, then what interventions should be tried?

5. Now that her children are all in school, she would like to return to the workforce as an accountant. She asks about workplace adaptations.

6. You perform a SI joint injection on her. Two weeks later, you learn that the methylprednisolone you injected into her has been recalled by the pharmaceutical company because it was contaminated with *Staphylococcus*. How would you explain this to her?

CASE 3: LOW BACK PAIN

Answers

1. First ask about "red flags": fevers, history of cancer, progressive weakness, and bowel or bladder incontinence. Next, further define the character of the pain. Ask about aggravating and alleviating factors. What is the impact on her function?

2. First inspect for kyphoscoliosis. Palpate over the spinous processes, paraspinals, SI joint, and trochanteric and ischial bursae. Test range of motion. Specific tests for common etiologies of back pain should be performed:
   - Radicular pain: Straight leg raising, femoral stretch, neurologic exam.
   - Facet cause: Facet loading, tenderness with palpation of the lumbar paraspinal area.
   - Sacroiliac (SI) joint pain: Tenderness to palpation of SI joint and provocative testing:
     a. Gaenslen (Figure 9.1)
     b. FABER / Patrick's test
     c. ASIS distraction (supine)
     d. Sacral compression (side lying)

3. An x-ray of the pelvis is indicated (anteroposterior angled and bilateral oblique views of the sacroiliac joints). MRI is not warranted and would result in lost points. Lab work should include HLA-B27 and ESR to exclude inflammatory sacroiliitis.

4. Therapy includes core strengthening, stretching (specifically of the hamstrings), strengthening of the legs and gluteus group, manual therapy, and modalities (ultrasound, iontophoresis, electrical stimulation). Aquatherapy can be considered. If conservative management is not helping or tolerated, an SI joint steroid injection may be helpful. If the relief is only temporary, prolotherapy or medial branch cauterization might also be considered. Fusion of the SI joint is a last-resort procedure.

5. Her future employer would be required to make reasonable accommodations under the Americans with Disabilities Act. One accommodation she could ask for is a standing frame for her desktop computer, allowing her to alternate between sitting and standing while working.

6. You need to call her and explain the facts of the situation. Ask her if she has experienced any ill effects. Tell her of whatever guidelines have been issued regarding monitoring and treatment. If she asks about legal action, you should advise her that you are not an attorney, but she may want to ask for advice from one. You should neither encourage nor discourage legal action.

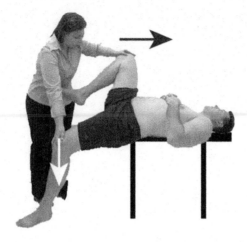

Figure 9.1 Gaenslen's maneuver.

BIBLIOGRAPHY

Barr KP, Harrast MA. Low back pain. In: Braddom R, ed. *Physical Medicine and Rehabilitation.* 4th ed. Philadelphia, PA: Elsevier;2011:871-911.

Cohen SP, Chen Y, Neufeld NJ. Sacroiliac joint pain: a comprehensive review of epidemiology, diagnosis and treatment. *Expert Rev Neurother.* January 2013; 13(1):99-116.

Nguyen TH, Randolf DC. Nonspecific low back pain and return to work. *Am Fam Physician.* 2007;76(10):1497-1502.

CASE 4: GENERALIZED MUSCULOSKELETAL PAIN

A 25-year-old woman presents with a 2-month history of pain in the neck, shoulders, back, and hips. She has no significant past medical history, and has had no trauma.

Questions

1. What more do you want to know about her history?

2. She has generalized achy pain. There are no radicular symptoms and no joint swelling. Pain interrupts her sleep. She gets no exercise. What physical exam elements are important?

3. What is the differential diagnosis, and what diagnostic testing is appropriate?

4. She has no evidence of inflammatory arthritis on her labs. She has a normal MRI of the brain and cervical spine. What are key elements of the treatment plan?

5. She states that exercise just makes her worse. Explain to the patient the importance of exercise for this diagnosis.

6. She tells you she wants to apply for Social Security disability. How should you respond?

CASE 4: GENERALIZED MUSCULOSKELETAL PAIN

Answers

1. You should question the patient about the character of the pain, exacerbating and relieving factors, radiation, arthralgias, numbness, weakness, and bowel and bladder symptoms. You should ask about sleep, exercise, and vocational and avocational interests. You should ask about past medical and family history.

2. Joints should be examined for synovitis and range of motion. A spine exam including Hoffman's and Spurling's tests should be performed. A thorough neurologic exam should include a check of motor and sensory impairments, reflexes, and balance. A tender point exam should be performed (Figure 9.2).

3. The differential diagnosis for diffuse axial pain in a young person includes cervical spine disease, Arnold Chiari malformation, myositis, inflammatory arthritis, multiple sclerosis, and fibromyalgia (FM). FM is a diagnosis of exclusion. Testing should include an autoimmune profile, CK, and MRI of the c-spine and brain.

4. She likely has FM. Treatment focuses on improving sleep and gradual increase in exercise. Medications effective for FM include pregabalin, gabapentin, and serotonin-norepinephrine reuptake inhibitors (SNRIs). The combination of pregabalin and duloxetine has been shown to be more effective than either alone. Secondary medications include tricyclic antidepressants (TCAs) and cyclobenzaprine. Sleep medication, particularly over-the-counter agents such as melatonin or diphenhydramine, may be helpful. Opioids and NSAIDs are generally not effective for FM and should be avoided.

5. First explain the scientific evidence for exercise in FM in lay terms. Behavioral interviewing would be helpful. Engage her in readiness for change, ask about barriers to exercise, and explain how she could overcome these barriers.

6. Social Security Disability has a very high threshold for qualification. She would need to demonstrate that she is unable to perform any work, irrespective of occupation. Most people with FM are able to work at least sedentary jobs. She would likely get rejected.

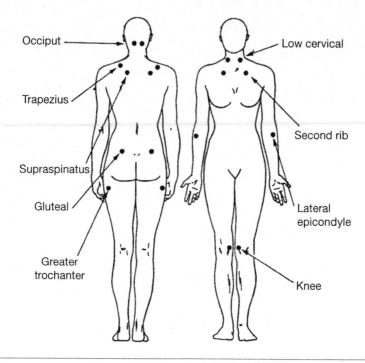

Figure 9.2 Fibromyalgia tender points.

BIBLIOGRAPHY

Abeles AM, Pillinger MH, Solitar BM, Abelas M. Narrative review: the pathophysiology of fibromyalgia. *Ann Intern Med.* 2007;146:726.
Goldenberg DL. Diagnosis and differential diagnosis of fibromyalgia. *Am J Med.* 2009;122(suppl):14-21.
Hauser W, Bernardy K, Arnold B, et al. Efficacy of multicomponent treatment in fibromyalgia syndrome: a meta-analysis of randomized controlled clinical trials. *Arthritis Rheum.* 2009;61:216-224.

CASE 5: CHRONIC HAND PAIN

A 35-year-old man fractured his left distal radius and ulnar in a fall 6 weeks ago. Upon removing the cast, his hand is exquisitely swollen, painful, and tender. Figure 9.3 shows its appearance.

Questions

1. What more do you want to know about his history and physical exam?

2. He has no relevant past medical history. He has diffuse allodynia and hyperalgesia in his hand. It is cool. There is hair loss and nail bed changes. What is the differential diagnosis? What diagnostic testing should be ordered?

3. Explain his diagnosis to him in lay terms.

4. Compartment pressures are normal. The patient could not tolerate EMG/NCS. X-ray shows a well-healed fracture but diffuse osteopenia of the hand. What is the treatment plan?

5. The fall occurred at work. He is a fast order chef. What obligations does his employer (or workers compensation insurer) have in terms of his rehabilitation and compensation?

CASE 5: CHRONIC HAND PAIN

Answers

1. How did the fracture occur? What is the character of the pain? Does he have involvement of any other joints? Does he have any significant past history?

2. Differential diagnosis includes compartment syndrome, non-union, nerve injury, and complex regional pain syndrome (CRPS). Compartment pressures should be checked urgently. Electrodiagnostic testing can be helpful if tolerated. X-rays should be obtained to look at fracture healing as well as osteopenia, which can be seen in severe CRPS.

3. Using eighth-grade level language, explain how CRPS is a misfiring of nerve impulses from the limb to the brain. Explain what is meant by vasomotor changes—swelling and temperature changes.

4. He likely has CRPS. A stellate ganglion block is the best initial treatment in acute onset upper limb CRPS. Neuropathic pain medicines such as gabapentin or SNRIs may help. Tricyclic antidepressants (TCAs) may also be helpful. The role of corticosteroids is unclear, but a short course might be tried. Physical or occupational hand therapy can include contrast baths, fluidotherapy, compression wraps, desensitization techniques, range of motion, and strengthening as tolerated. Early return to activity is thought to be helpful.

5. The employer is responsible for providing not only medical treatments but comprehensive rehabilitation including vocational services not typically covered by medical insurance. In addition, the employer must provide compensation until the patient can return to his old job. If the employee is unable to return to his previous job (permanent disability), then the employer must provide re-training for other work, or pay a permanent disability reward based on his level of impairment and his previous income.

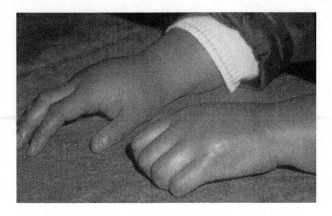

Figure 9.3 Complex regional pain syndrome.

BIBLIOGRAPHY

Bussa M, Guttilla D, Lucia M, et al. Complex regional pain syndrome type I: a comprehensive review. *Acta Anaesthesiol Scand*. 2015;59(6): 685-697.

Freedman M, Greis AC, Marino L, et al. Complex regional pain syndrome: diagnosis and treatment. *Phys Med Rehabil Clin N Am*. 2014;25(2):291-303.

Harden RN, Oaklander AL, Burton AW, et al. Complex regional pain syndrome: practical diagnostic and treatment guidelines. 4th edition. *Pain Med*. February 2013;14(2):180-229.

CASE 6: NECK AND HAND PAIN

A 52-year-old, right-handed man was referred to your clinic by his primary care provider. He complains of neck and right hand pain, as well as numbness and tingling in the right forearm and hand. His primary care provider prescribed him tramadol 50 mg PO TID and gave him a referral to physical therapy. He went to one session of physical therapy, but it made his symptoms worse.

Questions

1. What other information would you like to know about the history of his condition?

2. His symptoms have come and gone over the years, but became much worse when suddenly, at work as a mechanic, he felt a sharp, shooting pain down his arm. His pain is in the lateral half of his hand and fingers and up his lateral forearm. No recent injuries and no history of neck or carpal tunnel surgery are reported. He is having a hard time gripping and lifting with his right hand and arm and hasn't been able to go to work. He hasn't noticed any gait, bladder, or bowel changes. He has no fevers, recent weight loss, or history of cancer. His vital signs are within normal limits. What is important to do on physical exam?

3. He has decreased sensation in the C6 and C7 distribution, he has 4/5 strength of the finger abductors and wrist extensors, his brachioradialis deep tendon reflex is absent on the right, the Hoffman's test is negative, a Babinski test causes downgoing of the toes, right-sided Spurling's maneuver causes shooting pain from the neck into the arm, Phalen's test is negative, Tinel's test is negative at the wrist and elbow, his neck range of motion is normal, and there is no obvious neck deformity or tenderness to palpation of his neck. What is your differential diagnosis?

4. What tests would be appropriate to order to confirm your diagnosis?

5. Cervical x-rays show multilevel degenerative changes and narrowing of the disc space at C6-7, without any instability. Cervical MRI shows a C6-7 posterior lateral disc bulge with right-sided C6-7 neural foraminal narrowing (Figure 9.4). NCS/EMG, if ordered, reveals a C6-7 radiculopathy. You diagnose him with cervical radiculopathy. What are his options for treatment?

6. He asks for a physician work release. Would a work release be appropriate for his particular case?

7. He is resistant to returning to PT. Counsel him about the importance of this.

CASE 6: NECK AND HAND PAIN

Answers

1. Additional information includes onset of symptoms (gradual vs. sudden), exact location of pain, aggravating/alleviating factors, history of trauma, any history of neck/arm surgery, any associated weakness, any associated bladder or bowel dysfunction, any fevers, and any history of cancer.

2. Test for sensation in the affected limb, manual muscle testing, deep tendon reflexes, Hoffman's test, Babinski test, Spurling's maneuver, Phalen's maneuver, Tinel's test at the wrist, cervical range of motion, and inspection and palpation of the cervical spine.

3. The differential diagnosis involves cervical radiculopathy, cervical stenosis, brachial plexopathy, peripheral neuropathy (including entrapment neuropathies), and forearm tendinopathy.

4. Cervical spine x-rays (including flexion and extension views to look for instability) would be appropriate immediately if there is any history of trauma. A cervical MRI without contrast (contrast if cancer or infection is likely) is appropriate because of his subjective and objective neurologic deficit (weakness). Electromyography and nerve conduction study (EMG/NCS) could be ordered if there is a need to discern between spinal causes versus a peripheral cause such as carpal tunnel.

5. Ice/heat and massage are used for symptom management. NSAIDs (if no medical contraindications) can be prescribed. An oral steroid taper (e.g., Medrol Dose Pak) can be helpful to minimize inflammation and reduce pain while the patient is undergoing workup or conservative treatment. Neuropathic medications (such as gabapentin, pregabalin, tricyclic antidepressants, duloxetine) can help to treat the neuropathic component of pain. Opioids can help reduce pain, aid in sleep, and increase function (short-term only for severe pain and loss of function). Physical therapy can often help resolve radicular pain and is typically considered first-line treatment (manual treatment, modalities, traction, range of motion exercises). Cervical epidural steroid injections can decrease pain and may be indicated in this case of an identifiable cause of cervical radicular pain. Surgical referral would be appropriate and indicated if the patient does not respond to conservative treatment and has ongoing or worsening weakness.

6. A work release may be appropriate. We know he works as a mechanic and has been unable to perform his duties due to pain and weakness. Although he may not be able to perform his mechanic duties, it is important for him to explore whether or not his employer has opportunities for restricted work duties before fully relieving him of work. Patients who continue to stay at work or only take a short time off are more likely to return to work.

7. Explain how physical therapy is often painful the first few sessions, but provides longer term relief. In most cases, surgery can be avoided. The modalities and traction may reduce muscle spasm and pain. The exercises can strengthen muscles and stabilize the spine.

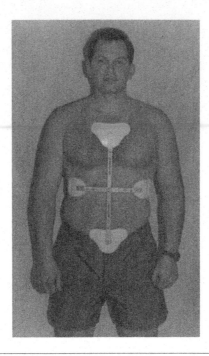

Figure 9.4 Cervical spine MRI revealing a C6-7 posterior lateral disc bulge.

BIBLIOGRAPHY

Bono CM, Ghiselli G, Gilgert TJ, et al. North American Spine Society evidence-based clinical guidelines for multidisciplinary spine care diagnosis and treatment of cervical radiculopathy from degenerative disorders. *N Am Spine Soc.* 2010. Available at: https://www.spine.org/ResearchClinicalCare/QualityImprovement/ClinicalGuidelines.aspx.

Bronstein AD, Macaulay SE, Singh RB, Cole AJ.Neurologic and musculoskeletal imaging studies. In: Braddom RL, ed. *Braddom's Physical Medicine and Rehabilitation.* 3rd ed. Philadelphia, PA: Elsevier;2007:125-150.

DePalma MJ, Slipman CW. Common neck problems. In: Braddom R, ed. *Physical Medicine and Rehabilitation.* 4th ed. Philadelphia, PA: Elsevier;2011:787-815.

CASE 7: LOW BACK PAIN IN MIDDLE-AGED WOMAN

A 49-year-old, left-handed female presents to your clinic with low back pain. She states that she has had the pain for years and it has gradually gotten much worse. In the past, it would come and go over the period of a few days. Now it is more persistent on a daily basis, especially in the morning and when she stays in any position for too long.

Questions

1. What other information would you like to know about her condition?

2. Her pain is located over the low back (lumbar) area. She does not recall having any pain or numbness going down the thighs or legs, nor any weakness to report. Her pain can range from a 2/10 to 9/10. It tends to be worse after rest or when going from a bent over position to standing. She does not have any history of trauma, surgery, or cancer. She does not have any bowel or bladder incontinence, nor does she report any fevers. What physical exam tests would be important to aid in diagnosis?

3. Her strength, sensation, reflexes, and gait are all within normal limitations. A Babinski test reveals downgoing of the toes bilaterally. She has a mild degree of lumbar scoliosis, mild pain to palpation of the lumbar paravertebral muscles, and worsening pain with extension maneuvers of the lumbar spine. FABER test does not reveal worsening pain and there is no pain over the sacroiliac joints. What is your differential diagnosis?

4. If the patient has failed conservative treatment before seeing you, what radiographic studies could aid in confirming diagnosis? Assuming no contraindications to the study, if imaging was ordered, what study would be the most appropriate given her lack of neurologic signs and symptoms?

5. A lumbar PA and lateral x-ray reveals lumbosacral spondylosis with moderate to severe facet joint arthropathy. What options for treatment does she have? Apart from basic conservative measures and pharmacological treatment, what is the next best treatment option for this patient?

6. Explain RFA to the patient in lay terms.

7. She returns to clinic after attending only one physical therapy session. She states that she cannot afford the co-pay on her insurance. She is, however, highly motivated to exercise. What options might she have?

CASE 7: LOW BACK PAIN IN MIDDLE-AGED WOMAN

Answers

1. Other relevant information includes the exact location of pain (any radiating symptoms [i.e., into the thighs/legs]), intensity of pain, aggravating/alleviating factors, history of trauma or back surgery, any associated weakness, any associated bladder or bowel dysfunction, any fevers, and any history of cancer.

2. Exam should include sensation of lower limbs, manual muscle testing, deep tendon reflexes, Babinski test, inspection and palpation of the lumbar spine and sacrum, range of motion of the lumbar spine, straight leg raising, facet joint loading, and special sacroiliac joint tests.

3. Differential diagnosis includes lumbar facet arthropathy, degenerative intervertebral disc disease (annular tear), lumbar myofascial pain, vertebral compression fracture, lumbar spondylolisthesis/spondylolysis, and sacroiliac joint arthropathy.

4. Possible studies are a lumbar x-ray, lumbar CT (only if an MRI is contraindicated), or lumbar MRI. It would be appropriate to attempt a course of conservative measures prior to obtaining imaging. A lumbar x-ray would be the most appropriate radiographic study (at least PA and lateral views; oblique views would aid in diagnosis of listhesis). An MRI should be reserved for patients with neurologic deficits, or for those with a high certainty of fracture, infection, or cancer, or failure of conservative treatment.

5. Conservative measures such as ice, heat, massage, acupuncture, chiropractic/osteopathic manipulation, and cognitive behavioral therapy are the next best treatments; NSAIDs are an option (if medically appropriate). Opioids should be used in the short term only for severe pain and loss of function. Physical therapy (manual treatment, modalities, core strengthening, and range of motion exercises) can also be beneficial. Facet joint injections or medial branch blocks with resultant RFA can be used if conservative management fails.

6. RFA deadens the nerve to the involved joint, reducing pain, often for a year or more when successful.

7. Exercise routines such as yoga or Pilates can be performed at home with instructional videos readily available on the Internet. These routines often have similar core strengthening exercises that a physical therapist might prescribe. She should be counseled about safety in doing these routines.

BIBLIOGRAPHY

Barr KP, Harrast MA. Low back pain. In: Braddom R, ed. *Physical Medicine and Rehabilitation*. 4th ed. Philadelphia, PA: Elsevier; 2011:871-911.
Chou R, Qaseem A, Snow V, et al. Diagnosis and treatment of low back pain: a joint clinical practice guideline from the American College of Physicians and the American Pain Society. *Ann Intern Med*. 2007;147:478-491.
Cohen SP, Raja SN. Pathogenesis, diagnosis, and treatment of lumbar zygapophysial (facet) joint pain. *Anesthesiology*. 2007;106(3):591-614.

CASE 8: OLDER PATIENT WITH MID BACK PAIN

A 74-year-old female comes to your office with a chief complaint of back pain for 3 weeks that has progressively gotten worse since the onset.

Questions

1. What other information would you like to know about her condition?

2. Her pain is located over the mid-to-lower back (thoracolumbar) area. She denies any weakness and pain or numbness going down the thighs or legs. Her pain ranges from a persistent 6-10/10. Lately it has been getting much worse. Her pain tends to get worse when bending forward. She does recall falling a few weeks back when rolling out of bed, but didn't have any immediate pain at the time; the pain started 2 days later. She does not have any history of surgery or cancer. She does not have any bowel or bladder incontinence and does not report any fever. What physical exam tests would be important to aid in diagnosis?

3. Her strength, sensation, reflexes, and gait are all within normal limitations. A Babinski test reveals downgoing toes bilaterally. She has a mild degree of lumbar scoliosis, and severe pain to palpation of the midline thoracolumbar junction. There is worsening pain with flexion maneuvers of the spine. What is your differential diagnosis?

4. What would be your next best step in diagnosis?

5. An MRI confirms your suspicion of a superior endplate vertebral compression fracture at L1. There is no neurologic compromise and no retropulsive fragments of bone, but there is a vertebral height loss of 20%. There is bone marrow edema seen on T2 images, indicating an acute-subacute fracture. Explain this to the patient in lay terms.

6. What are the important components of treatment?

7. Her fracture was the result of a fall. It is important for physicians to intervene to help prevent future falls. What additional questions should be asked?

CASE 8: OLDER PATIENT WITH MID BACK PAIN

Answers

1. Other relevant information includes the exact location of pain (any radiating symptoms; i.e., into the thighs/legs), intensity of pain, aggravating/alleviating factors, history of trauma, any history of back surgery, any associated weakness, any associated bladder or bowel dysfunction, any fevers, or any history of cancer.

2. Test the sensation of lower limbs, manual muscle testing, deep tendon reflexes, Babinski test, inspection and palpation of the entire spine, and range of motion of the lumbar spine.

3. The differential diagnosis includes vertebral compression fracture, discitis/osteomyelitis, spinal tumor, thoracolumbar spondylolysis/spondylolisthesis, and facet syndrome.

4. The next best step would be to obtain an MRI of the thoracic and lumbar spine. Based on her history of a recent fall, her age, gender, and severe pain with palpation of the spine in the midline, she most likely has a fracture. An MRI would be the diagnostic modality of choice to not only evaluate a potential vertebral compression fracture, but would also help define the age of the fracture and give important details for interventional decision making. An MRI would also help to evaluate for potential tumors (spinal metastasis) or an infection.

5. She has a compression fracture (partially crushed bone in her back). It is not unstable, and will likely heal in a few weeks. Surgery is rarely required.

6. Important components of treatment are pain control, maintenance of weight-bearing activity (walking aids if indicated), and potential fracture stabilization (bracing, vertebral augmentation such as vertebroplasty/kyphoplasty, or surgical treatment). Fracture stabilization is important to prevent worsening of the fracture while it is healing. At minimum a lumbar brace (lumbosacral orthosis [LSO]) should be ordered. A cruciform-anterior-spinal-hyperextension orthosis (CASH) brace helps place the lumbar spine in extension and prevents the potential damaging forces of flexion on a compression fracture and would be indicated (Figure 9.5). Indications for vertebral augmentation include: failure of pain control despite conservative treatment/bracing, worsening of fracture despite conservative treatment, minimal to no retropulsion of fracture, and no neurologic deficit due to the fracture. Surgery is indicated if there is more than a few millimeters of retropulsion of the fracture with failure of conservative treatment, or if there is any neurologic deficits from the fracture, and/or if the fracture has become vertebra plana (almost complete height loss of the vertebral body) with continued pain.

7. Prevention of future fractures is also important. Patients should have appropriate workup for potential causes of the fracture such as osteoporosis or tumors if indicated, and then receive appropriate treatment (such as bisphosphonates, calcium, and vitamin D for osteoporotic patients). A weight-bearing exercise program should ensue once the fracture is healed.

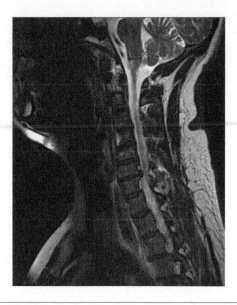

Figure 9.5 A cruciform-anterior-spinal-hyperextension orthosis (CASH).

BIBLIOGRAPHY

Huang C, Ross PD, Wasnich RD. Vertebral fracture and other predictors of physical impairment and health care utilization. *Arch Intern Med*. 1996;156(21):2469-2475.

Sekhadia M, Liu J. Osteoporosis, vertebroplasty, kyphoplasty. In: Benzon H, ed. *Essentials of Pain Medicine*. 3rd ed. Philadelphia, PA: Elsevier;2011:479-493.

Wong C, McGirt M. Vertebral compression fractures: a review of current management and multimodal therapy. *J Multidiscip Healthc*.2013;6:205-221.

CASE 9: ACUTE BACK PAIN

A 39-year-old male comes to your clinic because of 3 days of low back pain. He was referred to your clinic from the emergency department, where he went yesterday when his pain suddenly got much worse. They gave him some pain medicine and made him an appointment with you. He describes his pain as a deep ache in the low back and then it sometimes radiates up the low back on each side. It started when he was at work 3 days ago. He doesn't remember any specific event causing it. It gradually started to hurt and then got worse. He has never had any pain like this before.

Questions

1. What "red flag symptoms/signs" would you want to ask about to rule out the need for more immediate treatment or testing?

2. He denies all "red flag symptoms/signs." What would be the important components of the physical exam?

3. He has a normal exam except for some tenderness in the bilateral lumbar paraspinal muscles and decreased range of motion of the lumbar spine due to pain. What is the likely diagnosis?

4. What are the most important components of treatment for this condition?

5. The patient is relieved to hear that his pain is not likely a serious problem but wants to know what you are going to do to treat his symptoms. He has been using acetaminophen but it has not been helping much. What class of medication has shown good evidence for treatment of back pain? What risks come with using such a medication?

6. The patient wants something stronger than NSAIDs and acetaminophen for his pain. He is demanding "real" pain medicine. He says the other medication is not going to work and he cannot stand the pain anymore. How would you respond?

7. Describe how you might initiate a quality improvement project in your practice to reduce the amount of unnecessary radiographs ordered for acute back pain.

CASE 9: ACUTE BACK PAIN

Answers

1. Symptoms to consider include weakness, saddle anesthesia, bowel and/or bladder incontinence, fevers/chills, recent major unintentional weight loss/gain, history of cancer, major trauma, systemic prolonged steroid use, family history of inflammatory arthritis, or signs of more systemic disease (iritis, skin rashes, colitis, urethral discharge, etc.).

2. The physical exam should include a neurologic exam (strength, sensation, reflexes, primitive reflexes) and musculoskeletal exam (inspection, palpation, range of motion of the low back and sacroiliac joints, provocative tests, gait analysis).

3. The likely diagnosis is mechanical low back pain.

4. Treatment components include patient reassurance and education (this is a great opportunity to assure the patient his pain is likely to resolve and currently does not demonstrate any major serious concern), exercise/movement (the patient needs to continue to move either through a home program or with skilled therapy), and symptom control.

5. NSAIDs have been effective. Risks of major concern when using NSAIDs include GI discomfort and bleeding, renal dysfunction leading to high blood pressure, and cardiovascular risks.

6. This is a great opportunity to educate the patient about opioid pain medications and the risks of starting/using such medication. He should understand the risks of misuse, dependence, abuse, and the reasons for attempting non-opioid alternatives first. Opioid prescribing guidelines have been issued for prescribing opioids for chronic pain. While this patient currently has acute pain, the guidelines are appropriate whenever opioids are being considered, which include: using the lowest dose possible, only prescribing what is needed for the situation, frequent re-evaluation, documentation of functional benefits that validate the use of opioids, and potential urine drug screening to rule out the use of other controlled or illicit drugs that make prescribing opioids dangerous.

7. X-rays are indicated only for significant trauma or positive "red flags." You could start with a retrospective review of how often these guidelines are violated. Educate your colleagues and the patients on the guidelines, and prospectively see the impact. Continue with a PDSA (plan, do, see, and act) cycle by adapting various educational techniques to see which is the most effective.

BIBLIOGRAPHY

Barr KP, Harrast MA. Low back pain. In: Braddom R, ed. *Physical Medicine and Rehabilitation*. 4th ed. Philadelphia, PA: Elsevier;2011:871-911.

Bratton RL. Assessment and management of acute low back pain. *Am Fam Physician*. 1999;60(8):2299-2306.

Chou R, Qaseem A, Snow V, et al. Diagnosis and treatment of low back pain: a joint clinical practice guideline from the American College of Physicians and the American Pain Society. *Ann Intern Med*. 2007;147:478-491.

Nguyen TH, Randolf DC. Nonspecific low back pain and return to work. *Am Fam Physician*. 2007;76(10):1497-1502.

Van Duijvenbode I, Jellema P, van Poppel M, van Tulder MW. Lumbar supports for prevention and treatment of low back pain. *Cochrane Database Syst Rev*. 2008;16(2):CD001823.

10 Pediatric Rehabilitation

Sarah Korth, Frank Pidcock, Melissa Trovato, and Bryt Christensen

A mother brings her 15-month-old in for evaluation due to possible developmental delay. Records brought to the visit reveal the child was adopted from China at the age of 12 months. Prenatal and birth history is not available and medical/developmental information is limited. The mom does know the child was born full term. The child lived in an orphanage until adoption. Mom reports the child is not yet walking but is beginning to pull to stand. The child favors the right hand, which was noted at the orphanage.

Questions

1. What further questions would you ask?

2. How would you examine the patient?

3. The child is demonstrating a left hemiplegia. MRI of the brain is recommended to evaluate further for possible ischemic stroke or cerebral dysgenesis. The MRI reveals a middle cerebral artery infarction that is likely intrauterine or perinatal. The mom asks about the child's diagnosis. Based on the examination, what diagnosis are you considering and what testing do you recommend?

4. What therapies would you recommend for this child?

5. Mom asks, "Will my child walk and be normal like other kids?" What is your response?

6. As you are finishing the visit, the mother tells you she cannot afford the co-payments on the child's rehabilitation therapies. What options does she have?

CASE 1: DEVELOPMENTAL DELAY

Answers

1. Information regarding other developmental skills should be obtained including sitting, standing, holding onto a table or with assistance, cruising, grasp abilities of the hands, and what activities can be done with the left hand/arm. Information should be obtained about speech, oral motor skills, and eating. Are there vision or hearing issues? History of seizures? Any imaging or other evaluations that have been completed?

2. Physical exam findings include decreased active/functional use of the left upper extremity. Active movement of the wrist is noted for flexion and extension with reaching. The left hand tends to remain closed although passively range is full. Left lower extremity with decreased range at the ankle and mild tightness of the hamstring is noted, as well as two beats of clonus at the ankle. The child is able to sit independently and can come to sit, typically using the right extremity. When placed in supported standing the right foot is flat and the left is plantar flexed at initial foot contact but can relax to foot flat. The child speaks at least 5 to 10 words in Chinese and says 3 to 4 words in English.

3. Based on history, physical examination, and imaging, this child can be diagnosed with left hemiplegic cerebral palsy. The current definition of cerebral palsy is that it defines a group of disorders of the development of movement and posture, causing activity limitation, that are attributed to nonprogressive disturbances that occurred in the developing fetal or infant brain.

4. Constraint-induced movement therapy (CIMT) should be recommended in this child to facilitate spontaneous use of the left upper extremity, as well as functional finger movements. Physical therapy should be recommended to facilitate gross motor skills including standing and ambulation. As the child starts to do more weight bearing and ambulation, foot and ankle position should be monitored to determine the need for bracing to facilitate a normal gait pattern. Activities to encourage muscle strengthening and functional use are incorporated into play skills.

5. Children with hemiplegia due to perinatal ischemic stroke typically are independent ambulators and walk by age 2 if not sooner. Most kids develop functional use of the affected hand but for some fine motor skills may be impaired. Most have normal intelligence and participate in a regular school program and typical recreational activities. If upper extremity weakness causes functional impairments, accommodations can be made.

6. The child may be eligible for therapy in preschool.

BIBLIOGRAPHY

Ashwal S, Russman BS, Blasco PA, et al. Practice parameter: diagnostic assessment of the child with cerebral palsy: report of the Quality Standards Subcommittee of the American Academy of Neurology and the Practice Committee of the Child Neurology Society. *Neurology.* 2004;62(6):851-863.

Kitai Y, Haginoya K, Hirai S, et al. Outcome of hemiplegic cerebral palsy born at term depends on its etiology. *Brain Dev.* March 2016;38(3):267-273.

Rosenbaum P, Dan B, Leviton A, et al. Proposed definition and classification of cerebral palsy, April 2005. *Dev Med Child Neurol.* 2005;47:571-576.

Shin M, Kim H. Cerebral Palsy. In: *Knowledge Now.* 2017. Available at: https://now.aapmr.org/cerebral-palsy

CASE 2: TRAUMATIC BRAIN INJURY

A 6-year-old girl is admitted to a pediatric rehabilitation unit 3 months following a severe traumatic brain injury. The initial Glasgow Coma Scale score was 5 with prolonged loss of consciousness.

Questions

1. What key elements do you want to know from the history and examination that will shape the rehabilitation plan?

2. The child was in a coma for 7 days. She reports no pain. She is verbal but oriented to person only. She has no hemiparesis. She has progressed to a Rancho 4/5 level and is becoming agitated on the unit. She has kicked and bitten staff members. What strategies can be used to help manage the agitation, both nonmedication and medication? What are the risks/side effects associated with medication use?

3. The patient is very inattentive and is difficult to keep on task in therapy sessions. What recommendations can you provide to the team?

4. What are the developmental concerns regarding a patient of this age?

5. The patient has been in inpatient rehabilitation for 3 weeks and is no longer agitated but safety concerns persist due to inattention and short-term memory problems. What considerations would you have in planning for her discharge?

CASE 2: TRAUMATIC BRAIN INJURY

Answers

1. The following are important factors:
   a. Rancho level
   b. Duration of coma
   c. Ability to communicate
   d. Presence of pain
   e. Muscle strength
   f. Presence of contractures
   g. Cognitive exam
   h. Sensation
   i. Skin integrity
   j. Functional assessment

2. Strategies may include environmental changes as well as medications:
   a. Environmental strategies: Avoid overstimulation, maintain a quiet environment, have consistent staff treat the patient, provide frequent reassurance, and evaluate the impact of visitors and therapy and limit if causing agitation. Promote adequate sleep. Avoid use of restraints.
   b. Pharmacological strategies: Literature involving pediatric patients is limited.
      i. Benzodiazepines may be utilized but are not considered a good long-term solution. They may cause sedation and decreased concentration.
      ii. Beta blockers may be used until the intensity of agitation decreases. Side effects include bradycardia, orthostatic hypotension, and fatigue.
      iii. Anticonvulsants' side effects may include negative effects on cognitive and motor function.
      iv. Antipsychotics; adult studies have shown slow cognitive improvement or decreased cognitive return. The side effect list is long and can include weight gain, extrapyramidal symptoms, and neuroleptic malignant syndrome.

3. Strategies include:
   a. Pharmacological: There are limited studies; however, methylphenidate may be utilized and in several studies has shown improvement on test scores, as well as improved parent and teacher reports. Other stimulants have been clinically used as well.
   b. Minimize distraction by treating in a quiet room or area with less distractions.
   c. Give breaks as needed.
   d. Use preferred activities as a reward.

4. Family dysfunction and stress have been shown to increase following pediatric brain injury. In children the developmental stage may impact response to therapy and outcomes. Children with a brain injury are at increased risk for negative outcomes compared to adults. Injury during early childhood and elementary school may cause worse outcomes compared to children injured

as teenagers. When children are injured at a younger age it can impair their ability to gain the skills needed for later development. Milestones may not be reached that would allow the child to gain new skills. School reintegration is an important goal for the school-age child. As school progresses, demands increase in complexity. For children post brain injury who have difficulty with memory and executive functioning, the increased complexity of demands becomes more difficult to manage and they may fall behind their peers.

5. Discharge plans should include parental education. There should be a transition to a special education program in school with an individualized education plan. The child should receive ongoing physical, occupational, and speech therapy in school.

BIBLIOGRAPHY

Backeljauw B, Kurowski B. Interventions for attention problems after pediatric traumatic brain injury: what is the evidence? *PM&R.* 2014;6:814-824.

Cole W, Paulos S, Cole C, Tankard C. A review of family intervention guidelines for pediatric acquired brain injuries. *Dev Disabil Res Rev.* 2009;15:159-166.

Pangilinan P, Giacoletti-Argento A, Shellhaas R, Hurvitz EA, Hornyak JE. Neuropharmacology in pediatric brain injury: a review. *PM&R.* 2010;2:1127-1140.

Ponsford J, Janzen S, McIntyre A, et al. INCOG recommendations for management of cognition following traumatic brain injury, Part 1: posttraumatic amnesia/delirium. *J Head Trauma Rehabil.* 2014;29(4):307-320.

Rauh M, Aralis H, Melcer T, et al. Effect of traumatic brain injury among US service members with amputation. *JRRD.* 2013;50:161-172.

Suskauer S, Trovato M. Update on pharmaceutical intervention for disorders of consciousness and agitation after traumatic brain injury in children. *PM&R.* 2013;5:142-147.

CASE 3: BACK PAIN IN CHILDREN

An 11-year-old gymnast sees you for low back pain. She is very active in her sport and participates in local and regional competitions.

Questions

1. What information would you like to obtain on history and physical examination?

2. Pain is relatively sharp and worse with extension. On examination, she has tightness of her hamstrings and quads. There is localized tenderness in the left upper lumbar paraspinal musculature. Pain does not radiate into the lower limbs and strength is normal. What is your differential diagnosis? What diagnostic testing will you order? If an x-ray is ordered, what views would you order and why?

3. Lumbar x-ray (AP and lateral only) shows no abnormalities. MRI is normal. What is your next step? What instructions will you give to the patient?

4. Four weeks later the patient's flexibility has improved greatly, but she continues to report pain. What further imagining would you order?

5. Based on the evaluation to this point what is your next step?

6. In lay terms, explain the diagnosis to the patient and parents.

7. Her parents want to know, "When can she return to gymnastics?" How would you respond?

CASE 3: BACK PAIN IN CHILDREN

Answers

1. It is critical to assess the onset and duration of pain and if there were any acute trauma, as well as exacerbating or remitting factors. A lower limb neurologic examination should be completed.

2. Differential diagnosis includes spondylolysis, spondylolisthesis, lumbar strain, tumor, or infection. Tests include x-ray lumbar spine or MRI lumbar spine.

3. The next step is physical therapy directed at lower limb flexibility, core strengthening, and modalities for pain. Instructions include temporary removal from extension-based activities (removal from sport).

4. Imaging: MRI if not already ordered (normal) and a SPECT scan. The SPECT scan shows uptake at the bilateral L5 pars interarticularis. (This can be missed on MRI.) You may then order a thin cut CT through the area of uptake. CT shows bilateral L5 pars low-grade stress fracture (Figure 10.1).

5. Next step is Boston bracing for 3 months with continued follow-up; spine surgery if the fracture progresses.

6. This should be done in eighth-grade language. Her backbone is cracked, and may slip out of place.

7. This is a very serious injury that often results in major surgery should it progress. It would probably be better if she pursued a noncontact sport. She certainly should not return to gymnastics until the pars fracture is healed.

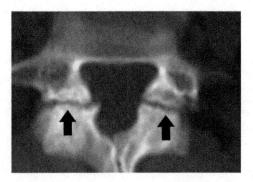

Figure 10.1 CT spondylolysis.

BIBLIOGRAPHY

Klein G, Mehlman CT, McCarty M. Nonoperative treatment of spondylolysis and grade I spondylolisthesis in children and young adults: a meta-analysis of observational studies. *J Pediatr Orthop.* 2009;29(2):146-156.
Leonidou A, Lepetsos P, Pagkalos J, et al. Treatment for spondylolysis and spondylolisthesis in children. *J Orthop Surg.* 2015;23(3):379-382.

CASE 4: SCOLIOSIS

An 11-year-old female presents to your office with her mother. The mother states that the patient was undergoing a routine physical examination by her family doctor for sports participation when she was found to have scoliosis. She was then referred to you for management.

Questions

1. What are some important factors to consider when collecting the patient history to help determine if the scoliosis is congenital, neuromuscular, or idiopathic?

2. She does not complain of any neurologic symptoms, has a normal birth history and childhood, and there is no relevant family history. Taking into consideration the referring diagnosis, what are the key components of her physical examination?

3. On exam you find no dysmorphic anatomy or any signs of congenital disease. She is neurologically intact with normal strength, sensation, and reflexes. Her spine has a rightward thoracolumbar curve and there is protrusion of the right rib cage and scapula. What diagnostic test(s) would you order? What would be the next step in management?

4. The radiographs show a 20 degree curvature. The mother asks why her daughter has a curved spine and if her daughter is going to need surgery. How would you respond? She then asks if her daughter will need a back brace or any additional treatments. How would you respond?

5. The patient expresses concern about her appearance. How can this be addressed?

CASE 4: SCOLIOSIS

Answers

1. Are there any pain or neurologic symptoms present (i.e., numbness, tingling, or weakness)? What is the patient's birth and pediatric milestone history (including growth)? Is there a family history of scoliosis or neuromuscular disease?

2. Key components include inspection/observation (any dysmorphic features or other signs of neuromuscular disorders; i.e., café-au-lait spots, dimpling of skin or tuft of hair over low back, long fingers or chest deformities); neurologic exam of cranial nerves and limbs (sensation, reflexes, and strength); musculoskeletal exam (inspection/palpation of spine and limbs, range of motion of spine, chest expansion, gait analysis).

3. Diagnostic tests include standing upright, plain radiographs of the spine (cervical, thoracic, and lumbar to measure degree of scoliosis), as well as pelvic radiograph (to measure Risser grade and better predict bone growth potential). If the curvature is <30 degrees, management is conservative with repeat x-rays in 1 year.

4. This is a great opportunity for patient and parent education regarding the patient's condition. There should be a discussion about the types of scoliosis (congenital, neuromuscular, and idiopathic), about how the most common cause is idiopathic, and how most cases do not require surgery. Also assure the parent that you will refer the patient to the appropriate surgical specialist if needed. Clarity of explanation and ability to give information in a compassionate, thoughtful, and caring manner are necessary. It is okay to tell the patient and the parent/caregiver that you do not know. Whether or not the patient will require bracing or any further treatment will be based on the degree of curvature, the potential for future growth, and the progression of the scoliotic curve over time. This is an opportunity to again educate the patient and parent in a clear, compassionate, and thoughtful manner.

5. Peer counseling can be beneficial if you have a support group in your area. Alternatively, psychological counseling may be needed, particularly if depressive symptoms develop.

BIBLIOGRAPHY

El-Hawary R, Chukwunyerenwa C. Update on evaluation and treatment of scoliosis. *Pediatr Clin North Am.* 2014;61(6):1223-1241.

Horne JP, Flannery R, Usman S. Adolescent idiopathic scoliosis: diagnosis and management. *Am Fam Physician.* 2014;89(3):193-198.

CASE 5: SPINA BIFIDA

A 14-year-old female with a S2 sacral level myelomeningocele comes into the examination room using Lofstrand crutches. She appears uncomfortable and complains of "tingly" feelings in her feet and increased fatigue. At her last visit 3 years ago, she did not require forearm crutches for short distance ambulation.

Questions

1. What questions would you ask her to further delineate the cause of her weakness? What are key elements of your physical exam?

2. You learn her weakness is localized to the lower extremities. This began about 10 months ago following her last visit to Multidisciplinary Spina Bifida Clinic. She was scheduled to return in 6 months but missed that appointment. She reports that her back aches especially after a busy day at school. She also states that her feet "look different." No fevers, headaches, diplopia, emesis, or lethargy is reported. She does have shunted hydrocephalus that has never required a revision. Vital signs are normal. She has no cranial nerve deficits. Vocal quality and volume is unchanged. Examination of the lower extremities shows left knee flexion is weaker than right. Foot inversion is weak on both sides. There is a calcaneo-valgus appearance of the foot. What is your differential diagnosis for her weakness?

3. What diagnostic tests are indicated?

4. Her MRI of the spine shows tethering of the cord at T11 to L1. What treatment would you recommend and what would you tell the patient and family?

5. Explain tethering of the cord in lay terms to the patient and family.

6. The reason she has not seen you in 3 years is that she missed her annual appointments in the spina bifida clinic. How would you address this with the patient and family?

CASE 5: SPINA BIFIDA

Answers

1. Does she have a ventricular shunt? Does she have headaches, lethargy, diplopia, or unusual emesis? Is there a change in her bladder and/or bowel routine? Has she gained weight? A thorough neuromusculoskeletal exam would include cranial nerve exam, sensation, strength, and any deformities in her lower limbs.

2. Differential diagnosis includes shunt malfunction, tethered cord, syringomyelia, compressive bone abnormalities, weakness secondary to weight gain, and deconditioning.

3. Testing includes brain imaging CT or MRI, full spine MRI, spine x-rays or CT, and urodynamic testing. CT or MRI of the head is required to rule out obstructive hydrocephalus. In the absence of a shunt or evidence of a working shunt, an MRI of the entire spine should be performed. Other studies could include spine x-rays or spine CT to look for bony abnormalities and to assess for scoliosis. Manual muscle testing and urodynamic testing should also be performed to document any changes and to provide a presurgical baseline.

4. Referral should be made to a neurosurgeon. Since almost all patients with spina bifida have some evidence of tethering on MRI, clinical judgment that includes clear evidence of deterioration in function is required before surgical untethering. All previous neuroimaging studies should be brought to the appointment. Symptomatic tethering can occur at any time throughout life.

5. In eighth-grade language, explain that the cord has become tangled. Treatment is usually surgical. Be careful not to be too scary in your language, and emphasize that this is treatable when caught early.

6. Deterioration of function is more difficult to reverse the longer the tethering is untreated. It is important not to miss scheduled appointments to the Spina Bifida Program. One should not be judgmental and should ask why the patient missed the appointments. Did the patient refuse? Did the family lose medical insurance? Was transportation a problem?

BIBLIOGRAPHY

Bui CJ, Tubbs RS, Oakes WJ. Tethered cord syndrome in children: a review. *Neurosurg Focus*. 2007; 23(2):1-9.

Dicianno BE, Kurowski BG, Yang JMJ, et al. Rehabilitation and medical management of the adult with spina bifida. *Am J Phys Med Rehabil*. 2008;87:1026-1050.

McDonald CM, Jaffe KM, Mosca VS, et al. Ambulatory outcome of children with myelomeningocele: effect of lower-extremity muscle strength. *Dev Med Child Neurol*. 1991;33(6):471-472.

CASE 6: PROGRESSIVE WEAKNESS IN A CHILD

A 5-year-old boy is brought to a pediatric PM&R clinic. His mother says he developed difficulty walking about 1 year ago. Otherwise, she had a normal pregnancy, and the patient walked normally until about 1 year ago. All vaccinations are up to date.

Questions

1. What questions would you ask before planning for further diagnostic workup?

2. The mother says the patient uses his hands to stand up from the ground. The decline in strength started about 1 year ago. His sister is 2 years older and healthy. The mother states she was adopted, and does not know if anyone in her family had neurologic disorders. What are the important physical findings and diagnostic workup? List the differentials as well.

3. An electrodiagnostic study showed normal sensory conduction results, but EMG shows small units with early recruitment patterns in proximal muscles. A muscle biopsy showed many atrophic myofibers with extensive necrosis and intermysial fibrosis. A further genetic workup reveals a mutation in the dystrophin gene. What is the prognosis? What is the plan for medical and rehabilitative management?

4. Five years later, the patient comes back to your clinic, and his mother is concerned about his poor academic performance. Per his mother, he was an A student, but since the new semester, he appears tired all the time and is seen sleeping during the class. What is your approach to this problem?

5. Fifteen years later, the patient comes back to your clinic after having fallen off from a bed during transfer. He is complaining of chest pain. He is currently living in a group home, and is dependent with all aspects of activities of daily living. On inspection, there are multiple bruises in the chest and trunk, and some of them appear to be old. What would you do?

CASE 6: PROGRESSIVE WEAKNESS IN A CHILD

Answers

1. Questions include time course/progression of symptoms; distribution of sensory symptoms, if any; pattern of muscle weakness; developmental delay; family history; and any musculoskeletal pain.

2. Items to evaluate are deep tendon reflexes; manual muscle testing; sensory exam; gait analysis; heart auscultation (to rule out murmur); general morphological inspection. Differentials include muscular dystrophy; spinal muscular atrophy; congenital myopathy; juvenile dermatomyositis; and mitochondrial myopathy.

3. This is a Duchenne muscular dystrophy, which is a progressive, fatal disease. He will likely be wheelchair-dependent during his teenage years, and his expected life span is 20 to 30 years. Given the progressive nature of the disease, early rehabilitative intervention is important. For example, a rollator can be considered for ambulation at this stage, but as he loses his ability to walk, a motorized wheelchair should be considered. Bracing is also needed to prevent scoliosis. In addition, he can be started on prednisone to delay the progression of motor weakness, after discussion with his family regarding potential benefits and risks.

4. Careful physical examination and medication history is important. Day-time narcolepsy is an early sign of respiratory distress due to reduced vital capacity, and history of sleep apnea should be obtained. If needed, pulmonary function tests should be considered. Psychosocial aspects of his school life should be examined as he is undergoing adolescence with severe disability; symptoms of depression, his social life with peers, and a possibility of bullying should be addressed

   Physical exam of the chest, including inspection, palpation, and auscultation, is the first step to rule out any life-threatening conditions. If it appears that he has been neglected or abused at the group home, contacting Adult Protective Services should be considered. Communication with caretakers and family members should also be mentioned.

BIBLIOGRAPHY

Amato AA, Russell JA.. Muscular dystrophies. In: Amato AA, Russell JA, eds. *Neuromuscular disorders*. New York, NY: McGraw-Hill; 2008:chap 24.

Bushby K, Finkel R, Birnkrant DJ, et al. Diagnosis and management of Duchenne muscular dystrophy, part 1: diagnosis and pharmacological and psychosocial management. *Lancet Neurol.* 2010;9(1):77-93.

Kellogg ND, Committee on Child Abuse and Neglect, American Academy of Pediatrics. Evaluation of suspected child physical abuse. *Peds.* 2007;119(6):1232-1241.

11 Soft Tissue Impairments

R. Samuel Mayer

You are consulted on a 45-year-old woman with spastic diplegic cerebral palsy who was recently admitted to a nursing facility after her elderly parents were no longer able to care for her. She was ambulatory with forearm crutches until 3 years ago. She says her legs have become so bent up she can no longer stand on her own.

Questions

1. What further information do you want to know?

2. You learn that they now use a Hoyer lift at the nursing facility to get her out of bed. She does not get physical therapy there, as she is in custodial care. The nursing staff does not perform range of motion or stretching with her. She is currently on baclofen 10 mg three times daily, but cannot tolerate higher doses as it makes her confused. She has no splints. As a child she remembers having serial casting, and that it helped. She had no surgeries. She had botulinum toxin injections in the past but they did not help, and were discontinued. What are key elements in the physical exam?

3. Her upper limbs are normal. She has fixed contractures of her hips, knees, and ankles. Her hips have 10-degree flexion contractures, her knees have 45-degree flexion contractures, and her ankles have 5-degree flexion contractures. Deep tendon reflexes are absent at knees and ankles; Babinski is up bilaterally. Due to the severity of her contractures, you cannot assess her tone. She has no skin breakdown. What diagnostic testing is indicated?

4. X-rays of her hips show shallow acetabulum bilaterally, but no other abnormality; x-rays of knees and ankles are normal. What is your treatment plan?

5. Explain to the patient in lay terms her diagnosis and treatment.

6. She has no remaining benefits for physical therapy, and the nursing home administration refuses to pay for dynamic splints, which would cost approximately $1,000. How would you approach this?

CASE 1: CONTRACTURE

Answers

1. Questions include: How does this affect her function? What is her mobility like? What treatment has she received in the past or is currently receiving?

2. You would need to measure range of motion in the limbs. You would also assess tone, reflexes, and upper tract signs. You would look for pressure sores.

3. X-rays of her joints are needed to look for heterotopic ossification or other orthopedic abnormalities.

4. Treatment of her spasticity might include phenol injections or additional oral medications (dantrolene or tizanidine). She might be a candidate for an intra-thecal pump. However, treatment of her spasticity without treatment of the mechanical contracture will be futile. She will need some form of prolonged stretching, either with dynamic splints or serial casting.

5. Explain in eighth-grade language that her tendons have shortened due to chronic muscle spasms. You will try to relieve the spasms with the medica-tions or injections, and will need to do a prolonged stretch of the muscles with splints or casts.

6. If you have the skills, serial casting could be an option, but you would also need to make sure the facility's nursing staff is able to monitor this. Unfortunately, when a patient is in a custodial level of care, physical therapy is not a covered benefit by insurance. Durable medical equipment must be provided by the facility at their cost. You can try to advocate with the adminis-trator for the dynamic splints, emphasizing risk of pressure sores if untreated. This would be a quality issue for the nursing home, and they could get cited.

BIBLIOGRAPHY

Fergusson D, Hutton B, Drodge A. The epidemiology of major joint contractures: a systematic review of the literature. *Clin Orthop Relat Res.* 2007;456:22-29.

Katalinic OM, Harvey LA, Herbert RD, et al. Stretch for the treatment and prevention of contractures. *Cochrane Database Syst Rev.* September 8, 2010;2(9):CD007455.

Moriyama H, Tobimatsu Y, Ozawa J, et al. Amount of torque and duration of stretching affects correction of knee contrac-ture in a rat model of spinal cord injury. *Clin Orthop Relat Res.* 2013;471(11):3626-3636.

CASE 2: PRESSURE SORE

A 28-year-old man with tetraplegia returns to the clinic for the first time in 5 years. He tells you he has not had medical problems and has come back to have the proper documentation for a manual wheelchair. Your physical exam is significant for C7 AIS A with a Zone of Partial Preservation to T1 for motor and sensory bilaterally.

Questions

1. He has pressure sores on his buttocks (Figure 11.1). What key elements do you want to know about the pressure sores?

2. He has two clean pressure injuries that do not have signs of infection located at his bilateral ischial tuberosities that are Stage III and about 7 cm in the largest diameter. He has had them for about 3 months and is treating them himself with wet to dry dressing changes. What do you need to know from his ROS, functional, and social history?

3. He is in the wheelchair all day and performs weight shift whenever he remembers. He uses a sliding board to transfer independently. He often voids in a diaper for bowel and bladder because transfers are difficult. He smokes 1 pack of cigarettes per day. What is the treatment plan for healing the pressure ulcers?

4. He returns in 6 months with the ischial wounds healed, but has now developed sacral and right greater trochanter wounds that are being managed by the wound care team. What durable medical equipment should be prescribed?

5. In lay terms, explain to him the importance of pressure relief.

6. An insurance reviewer requests a peer-to-peer conversation regarding the durable medical equipment you recently prescribed, specifically the power wheelchair with tilt-in-space feature and cushion with pressure mapping. How do you justify the wheelchair?

CASE 2: PRESSURE SORE

Answers

1. You would want to know the, location, stage, tunneling, signs of infection, duration, and treatment.

2. You would need to know the constitutional information (weight gain, nutritional status), method of transfers, sitting time, weight shifts, bowel program, bladder program, and smoking history. Smoking increases risk of pressure sores.

3. Treatment involves referral to the wound care team, home health care referral for the wound care, no more sitting upright until pressure ulcers heal, smoking cessation, and a bowel and bladder program in bed.

4. Durable medical equipment prescribed should include a power wheelchair with tilt-in-space feature, cushion with pressure mapping, and air mattress.

5. Using eighth-grade language, explain that moving pressure off the buttocks every 2 hours is essential. Explain how his limited sensation impacts this.

6. Mobility in tetraplegia is challenging. Transfers are impossible to different elevations. The patient requires a power wheelchair with adjustable heights to help with his transfers. Likewise, weight shift is not possible with the weight gain and given the history of pressure injury; he requires a tilt-in-space feature.

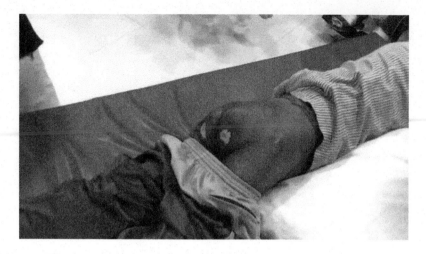

Figure 11.1 Stage 3 gluteal pressure sore.

BIBLIOGRAPHY

Bergstrom N, Horn SD, Smout RJ, et al. The National Pressure Ulcer Long-Term Care Study: outcomes of pressure ulcer treatments in long-term care. *J Am Geriatr Soc.* 2005;53:1721.

Chen Y, Devivo MJ, Jackson AB. Pressure ulcer prevalence in people with spinal cord injury: age-period-duration effects. *Arch Phys Med Rehabil.* 2005;86(6):1208-1213.

Consortium for Spinal Cord Medicine Clinical Practice Guidelines. Pressure ulcer prevention and treatment following spinal cord injury: a clinical practice guideline for health-care professionals. *J Spinal Cord Med.* 2001;24 (suppl 1):S40-S101.

12 Spinal Cord Injury

Argyrios Stampas

CASE 1: TRAUMATIC QUADRIPLEGIA WITH DECREASED HAND FUNCTION

A 35-year-old man with traumatic cervical spinal cord injury sustained 5 years ago in a motor vehicle accident status postcervical decompression and fusion presents to your clinic with complaints of loss of hand function. His physical exam from last year was significant for C7 AIS C.

Questions

1. What key elements do you want to know from his history? What do you need to ask about in your review of systems?

2. The patient tells you that he has been having progressive loss of strength over 2 to 3 months in his bilateral hands, affecting his manual wheelchair propulsion over the past few months as well as his grip. He is also having hand and finger dysesthesias, and neck pain that feels like soreness. He denies changes in bowel and bladder function, and reports no falls or trauma. What is critical to do on physical exam?

3. Physical exam is significant for C5 sensory level with C7 motor level. The motor exam has not changed significantly from prior exams. Tinel's and Phalen's tests are equivocal bilaterally. What is the differential diagnosis of his progressive weakness? What diagnostic testing, if any, is indicated?

4. Cervical x-ray is negative for hardware failure and acute fracture, and MRI reveals no syrinx. EMG is significant for median neuropathy at the wrist. What intervention would help him?

5. Explain his diagnosis and treatment in lay terms.

6. He returns to clinic 1 month later and states that many of his symptoms have improved, but he continues to have difficulty propelling his manual wheelchair. How would you advise the patient?

CASE 1: TRAUMATIC QUADRIPLEGIA WITH DECREASED HAND FUNCTION

Answers

1. Over what time frame did the change occur? We need to know about sensory changes in the upper extremities, changes with his bowel program (constipation, accidents, etc.), changes with his bladder program (frequency, urgency, urinary tract infections, etc.), history of recent fall or trauma, and changes with neuropathic pain and/or paresthesia. Specific information is needed regarding the hand function loss. Review of systems should include constitutional issues (fevers, chills, and weight loss/gain), polydipsia, hunger, fatigue, and blurred vision (DMII symptoms).

2. Physical examination includes an American Spinal Cord Injury Association Impairment Scale exam to determine change in neurologic level, rectal exam, shoulder exam, and Phalen's and/or Tinel's test.

3. Differential diagnosis includes carpal tunnel syndrome, ulnar neuropathy, radiculopathy, hardware failure and cord/root impingement, syringomyelia, and peripheral neuropathy. A cervical x-ray is indicated to rule out hardware failure, MRI of the cervical spine to rule out syringomyelia, and a bilateral NCS/EMG to rule out radiculopathy. A peripheral neuropathy test should be performed.

4. Treatment includes occupational therapy consultation for learning to improve wrist positioning during activities of daily living and ergonomic wheelchair adjustments, education on ergonomic workspace, wrist/hand orthosis to be worn while sleeping, and gabapentin/pregabalin/amitriptyline/nortriptyline for neuropathic pain management. If he fails to improve with this, corticosteroid injection can be considered. Surgery would be a last resort, especially since it might limit his ability to transfer independently during postoperative recovery.

5. With eighth-grade language, explain that carpal tunnel syndrome is a pinching of the nerve in the wrist that can weaken the hand muscles and cause pain. It comes from excessive pressure, such as propelling the wheelchair or transferring.

6. He should be seen by a therapist and evaluated for smart-assist wheels. He would also benefit from outpatient therapy for strengthening. Weight loss would also make wheelchair propulsion easier.

BIBLIOGRAPHY

Tan W-H, Skelton F. Overuse injuries in disorders of the central nervous system. *Knowledge NOW.* 2013. Available at: http://me.aapmr.org/kn/article.html?id=28.

van Drongelen S, de Groot S, Veeger HEJ, et al. Upper extremity musculoskeletal pain during and after rehabilitation in wheelchair-using persons with a spinal cord injury. *Spinal Cord.* 2006;44:152-159.

CASE 2: POSTOPERATIVE PARESIS

A 56-year-old male presents to your clinic complaining of worsened weakness since his back surgery 3 weeks ago. He tells you that it was the third surgery on his lower back and he needed it because he was getting weak in his legs.

Questions

1. What key elements do you want to know about his preoperative symptoms and workup?

2. He tells you that his operation was on L2 and L3 because of weakness in his legs and back pain. An MRI showed disc disease and herniation at the L2-3 level. EMG was significant for bilateral L3 radiculopathy. What do you want to know about his postoperative course?

3. He had an uncomplicated surgery. Postoperatively he had profound weakness in his feet that improved somewhat. He had an indwelling catheter that was removed on day of discharge and, after a long time, he voided about 1 liter of urine. He is now often incontinent of bowel and bladder. What are the critical components of the physical exam?

4. Why is incontinence such an important issue?

5. Physical exam is significant for 4/5 strength in L2 and L3, and 1/5 strength in L4-S1 myotomes, reduced sensation in L2-S5 dermatomes, 1+ patellar reflexes and areflexic in Achilles reflex, positive deep anal pressure, no voluntary anal contraction, and no anal wink with pin prick. What is your assessment? What is the plan for bowel and bladder management?

6. He has followed your program and has not had bowel or bladder accidents. However, he is concerned about his sexual function and wants to know what can be expected with treatment, if possible. What do you advise him about this?

CASE 2: POSTOPERATIVE PARESIS

Answers

1. Questions include: What were the indications for surgery (symptoms were pain, weakness, sensory loss, bowel or bladder incontinence, instability)? What vertebral levels were involved in the surgery? What previous workup has he had including imaging and electrodiagnostics? What is his current bowel and bladder function?

2. Did he have complications (infections, deep vein thrombosis, hemorrhage)? What symptoms did he have postoperatively (weakness, sensation, bowel/bladder)? What was his discharge location (home, acute, or subacute rehabilitation)?

3. Critical components are manual motor testing in the bilateral lower extremities (BLE), sensory testing in the BLE, deep tendon reflexes in the BLE, rectal exam with pin and light touch, and observation of anal wink reflex.

4. Incontinence is socially very disconcerting to patients. It can lead to skin breakdown. It is one of the most common reasons patients wind up in long-term facilities. The social and economic costs are enormous.

5. The assessment is L1 AIS C (conus medullaris syndrome) with lower motor neuron bowel and bladder. He should have a bowel program with promotility (senna, bisacodyl) and bulking (fiber) with an enema or manual disimpaction for daily bowel movement. Bladder will need urology follow up for urodynamics.

6. When discussing sexuality, it is useful to ask the patient about his or her perceptions, and to probe culturally what kind of detail the patient is comfortable discussing. Sildenafil (Viagra) is very efficacious for erectile dysfunction but not for ejaculation. He may have infertility because of this. Sperm donation with electro-ejaculation is possible.

BIBLIOGRAPHY

Gonzalez-Fernandez M. Bowel care medications. In: Gonzalez-Fernandez M, Friedman JD, eds. *Physical Medicine and Rehabilitation Pocket Companion.* Vol 1. 1st ed. New York, NY: Demos; 2011:326-329.

Podnar S, Trsinar B, Vodusek DB. Bladder dysfunction in patients with cauda equina lesions. *Neurourol Urodyn.* 2006;25(1):23-31.

Todd NV, Dickson RA. Standards of care in cauda equina syndrome. *Br J Neurosurg.* October 2016;30(5):518-522.

CASE 3: SPASTICITY

A 35-year-old male presents to your clinic with C5 AIS C spinal cord injury complaining of worsening spasticity over the past year. The spasms interfere with his transfers and have caused him to fall several times. He is taking baclofen 20 mg four times daily, and complains of fatigue from it.

Questions

1. What key questions do you have related to worsening spasticity?

2. The patient has not had noticeable differences with his sensation or strength. He has had more bladder accidents in between catheterizations and has had less production with his bowel program. What are the critical components of the physical exam?

3. His exam is stable with C5 AIS C. He has stool in his rectum and has decreased bowel sounds with a distended abdomen. Spasticity is 3/4 on the Modified Ashworth Scale for shoulder, elbow flexors and finger flexors, hip adductors, knee extensors and flexors, and ankle plantar- and dorsi-flexors. He has sustained clonus in upper and lower limbs. What imaging and/or laboratory analysis should be ordered and why?

4. After a few minutes, he returns having completed an abdominal x-ray that is significant for a large volume of stool and nephrolithiasis. What is the next course of management?

5. He returns to the clinic after successful lithotripsy and bowel cleanout. He continues to have spasticity for which he takes baclofen and he is concerned about the side effects of constipation and sedation. You added tizanidine, which made him orthostatic, and tried dantrolene but this made him feel weak all over. What other spasticity management would you recommend?

6. He does well with the baclofen pump trial. What psychosocial considerations are important to consider before placing the pump?

7. In lay terms, explain the risks and benefits of the baclofen pump to the patient.

CASE 3: SPASTICITY

Answers

1. Questions include: Are there changes in the strength, sensation, bowel, and/or bladder program? Does he have any inciting irritation, for example, urinary tract infections, pressure sore, fecal impaction, or infection?

2. Critical components include the ISNCSCI exam (sensory, motor, rectal), spasticity test (Modified Ashworth or Tardieu Scale), presence of clonus, abdominal exam, and skin exam for pressure sores.

3. Urinalysis with culture is ordered to rule out urinary tract infection. Abdominal x-ray is ordered to evaluate stool burden.

4. Aggressive bowel cleanout (magnesium citrate or lactulose) and Fleet enema to reduce stool burden are the next steps. Improve the daily bowel program. A urologist follow-up for nephrolithiasis is recommended. Add tizanidine and/or dantrolene for his spasticity.

5. He is likely a candidate for an intrathecal baclofen pump, as he has generalized spasticity uncontrolled by oral medications. He should have a trial dose of intrathecal baclofen and, if successful, a pump installed.

6. Follow-up with a baclofen pump is critical, as an empty pump can be a fatal occurrence from baclofen withdrawal. He must have transportation available to get to appointments, or a home care agency in his area that can do refills. He has to be able to understand the signs and symptoms of withdrawal and overdose. And he will need insurance coverage for not only the procedure but the continued refills as well.

7. In eighth-grade language, explain how the pump delivers the medicine directly to the fluid around the spinal cord and brain, requiring a much smaller dose and with fewer side effects. However, explain the risk of sudden withdrawal if the pump is not refilled or the system fails. Also explain the risk of infection and meningitis. Explain catheter problems, and possible pump failure. Stress the importance of follow-up.

BIBLIOGRAPHY

Adams MM, Hicks AL. Spasticity after spinal cord injury. *Spinal Cord.* 2005;43:577–586.

Francisco GE. The role of intrathecal baclofen therapy in the upper motor neuron syndrome. *Eur Med Phys.* 2004;40:131-143.

Wantanabe T. The role of therapy in spastic management. *Am J Phys Med Rehabil.* 2004;10(S):S45-S49.

CASE 4: AUTONOMIC DYSREFLEXIA

A 35-year-old male with C5 AIS A tetraplegia sustained in a motor vehicle collision 2 weeks ago is admitted to your inpatient rehabilitation unit. He has a tracheostomy and is on a ventilator at night, IV access in his right arm, and an indwelling Foley catheter. Nursing calls you immediately because of complaints of headache, flushing, and chills.

Questions

1. What key elements do you want to know about his physical exam?

2. His systolic blood pressure is 150/95 mmHg, pulse is 55. Otherwise, vitals are within normal limits. His Foley is not draining. What are the next steps in the management of this patient?

3. The Foley flushes and his systolic blood pressure drops to 120 mmHg. The patient and family are concerned and want to know what happened and, if untreated, what could be the consequences. What do you tell him?

4. He has another episode of autonomic dysreflexia a week later. His systolic blood pressure is now 180 mmHg. You discover an edematous, erythematous, ingrown toenail. The podiatrist can come this evening to treat the patient. What is the management in the interim?

5. He returns to your outpatient clinic 1 month after discharge. He tells you that he does not consistently get his bowel program because his wife works during the day and his teenage daughter is not comfortable doing it. He gets autonomic dysreflexia once or twice a week due to constipation. What are alternatives for him?

CASE 4: AUTONOMIC DYSREFLEXIA

Answers

1. Check vital signs (blood pressure, temperature, heart rate, respiration rate, pulse oximetry), penis, and drainage of Foley. One should do a rectal exam to exclude fecal impaction (done with lidocaine gel). Check for pressure sores and ingrown nails.

2. Apply a blood pressure cuff for monitoring, loosen clothing, sit the patient up, and flush the Foley.

3. You need to educate the family using lay terms. You need to explain how the spinal cord injury affects internal organs in addition to the arms and legs. Autonomic dysreflexia can lead to seizures, retinal hemorrhage, pulmonary edema, renal insufficiency, myocardial infarction, cerebral hemorrhage, and death. You need to explain the early warning signs such as flushing, sweating, and headache. You need to discuss how bowel, bladder, and skin care are important in preventing this.

4. Hold from therapy until blood pressure is controlled; monitor vitals q 2 hours, and administer analgesics if needed using fast-acting antihypertensive medications to control blood pressure (nitro paste, nitroglycerine sublingual, hydralazine, nifedipine, or captopril).

5. In some states, Medicaid will provide home health aides for several hours per day. Sometimes private insurance will provide this as well. Usually this is quite limited under Medicare. He may have to hire help, or alternatively, have his wife do the bowel program in the evenings when she is home.

BIBLIOGRAPHY

Christopher and Dana Reeve Foundation. *Autonomic Dysreflexia Pamphlets.* Available at: http://www.christopherreeve.org/site/c.mtKZKgMWKwG/b.4453413/k.5E2A/Autonomic_Dysreflexia.htm.
Garstang SV, Walker H. Cardiovascular and autonomic dysfunctions after spinal cord injury. In: Kirshblum S, Campagnolo DI, eds. *Spinal Cord Medicine.* 2nd ed. Philadelphia, PA: Wolters Kluwer Health/Lippincott Williams & Wilkins; 2011.
Krassioukov A, Warburton DE, Teasell R, et al. A systematic review of the management of autonomic dysreflexia after spinal cord injury. *Arch Phys Med Rehabil.* 2009;90(4):682-695.

CASE 5: CENTRAL CORD SYNDROME

An 85-year-old woman with central cord syndrome is on your inpatient rehabilitation service. She sustained a nonoperative spinal injury without fracture. She is wearing a Halo vest.

Questions

1. What are the focused exam findings pertinent to the care of those wearing a Halo vest?

2. Her rehabilitation course was uneventful and she was discharged to a skilled nursing facility. She returns to your clinic 12 weeks later. The Halo vest was removed by the spine surgeon, and she is now wearing a hard cervical thoracic orthotic (SOMI) brace. She tells you she has had a red area on her jaw that is worsening despite ointments. What are the pertinent exam findings related to her skin?

3. You tell her she has developed a pressure ulcer, make the proper adjustments on the collar, and educate her about pressure relief. She tells you she has had her neck in a Halo and in this brace for over 3 months and would like to remove it entirely. She is sick and tired of wearing this. How should you respond?

4. One month later, she was discharged home requiring minimum assistance for ambulation and maximum assistance for activities of daily living. Her jaw pressure ulcer has healed and the brace has been discontinued by her surgeon. She returns to the clinic to discuss options for regaining upper extremity function. What do you prescribe?

5. She is interested in a stem cell treatment she found on the Internet that is only available in Asia. She tells you that after stem cell infusion IV and 3 months of therapy costing $12,000, testimonials report excellent neurologic recovery. She wants your opinion. How should you advise her?

CASE 5: CENTRAL CORD SYNDROME

Answers

1. Pertinent exam findings include pin site inspection, loosening of pins, and skin exam beneath the vest.

2. Questions to ask include: Is it blanchable? Is the pressure from the hard collar at the site of erythema? Is the collar an appropriate size?

3. Express understanding about her frustration. Unfortunately, she should not remove the collar until cleared by the surgeon after imaging reveals satisfactory healing. She should get flexion/extension films of the cervical spine prior to her next visit with the spine surgeon. Premature removal of bracing can lead to further spinal cord compression from spinal instability.

4. Prescribe occupational therapy evaluations and therapy two or three times weekly, with upper limb functional electrical stimulation, robotics, wrist-hand orthotics, and assistive devices.

5. You should highly discourage this: There is no biological mechanism and no evidence for efficacy. Money can be spent on home exercise equipment and therapy.

BIBLIOGRAPHY

American Spinal Injury Association. *International Standards for Neurological and Functional Classification of Spinal Cord Injury—Revised 2011*. Atlanta, GA: ASIA; 2011.

Devivo MJ, Chen Y. Trends in new injuries, prevalent cases and aging with spinal cord injury. *Arch Phys Med Rehabil.* 2011;92(3):332-338.

Yang J, Gosai E, Avers S. Cervical, thoracic and lumbosacral orthoses. 2017. *Knowledge NOW.* Available at: https://now.aapmr.org/cervical-thoracic-and-lumbosacral-orthoses

13 Stroke Rehabilitation

J. George Thomas

CASE 1: POST-STROKE DEPRESSION

A 59-year-old female has been in the inpatient rehabilitation unit for 2 weeks after a left frontal ischemic stroke. Her nurse indicates that the patient has been showing a rather flat affect and her daily food intake has been poor for the past 2 days.

Questions

1. What would you like to know from your history and physical of the patient to assess these complaints?

2. The patient reports she feels like she'll never get better: "What's the point in going on like this?" She has poor sleep and appetite. She denies nausea, constipation, or diarrhea. Her physical exam is unchanged from admission. What are some screening tools that will help establish a diagnosis of poststroke depression?

3. Your evaluation of the stroke patient indicates that the patient had prestroke depression and is currently intermittently tearful during therapies along with significantly decreased appetite and some fatigue. What are the considerations for treatment of her poststroke depression?

4. The patient's family asks whether there are any risk factors for poststroke depression and its prognosis. What will you discuss regarding this with the family?

5. The patient and her family are devout Wahhabi Muslims, and are adamantly opposed to the use of antidepressants on religious grounds. How would you approach this?

CASE 1: POST-STROKE DEPRESSION

Answers

1. The physician should get a good review of systems to ensure that the patient has no physiologic problems (e.g., nausea, constipation) causing the loss of appetite. One should ask about vegetative signs of depression including mood, anhedonia (loss of interest in usual activities), change in sleep (insomnia or hypersomnia), and changes of appetite (anorexia or overeating). A depressed patient should always be questioned about suicidal ideation. The exam should include both a neurologic and abdominal exam.

2. There are self-report screening tools that help diagnose depression such as the Beck Depression Inventory (BDI), Hospital Anxiety and Depression Scale (HADS), Geriatric Depression Scale (GDS), and Visual Analog Mood Scale (VAMS). Observational scales include the Post-stroke Depression Rating Scale (PDQRS) and Stroke Aphasia Depression Questionnaire (SADQ-H 10 or 21). Poststroke depression is underdiagnosed in 50% to 80% of cases, and the physiatrist should have a protocol to assess every stroke patient for depression. As part of history taking and interview, one has to ask questions about difficulty with appetite, sleep, energy levels, or ability to concentrate. Poststroke depression can present as apathy (seen in 23% to 57% of stroke patients), in addition to expressed feelings of worthlessness or thoughts of death or suicide.

3. While counseling and psychotherapy have shown little efficacy early in poststroke depression, psychotherapy can be helpful with minor depression and with milder cognitive impairments. With apathy and lethargy in this patient, psychostimulants such as methylphenidate can be used first, followed by SSRIs. The most studied in poststroke depression treatment are citalopram, mirtazapine, and sertraline. Increasingly SNRIs such as venlafaxine and duloxetine are also being used. There is no evidence that one SSRI is better than another. The physiatrist has to balance out the benefits of using antidepressants versus the risk of seizures, cognitive effects, and falls.

4. The physiatrist should tell the patient's family that approximately one third of stroke patients do develop clinically significant depression at some point after the stroke. It is important to note that poststroke depression is not related to any character weakness on the patient's part, and may result from physiologic changes in the brain after stroke. Approximately 40% of the patients develop symptoms within 3 months of stroke. Many stroke patients can develop depression after discharge from the inpatient rehabilitation unit. Interestingly, most patients with major poststroke depression appear to recover significantly better than minor post-stroke depression (PSD) by 2 years after the stroke. There is controversy regarding the location of the left cortical and subcortical lesions as higher risk for depression. The level of disability (low Barthel index score), inadequate social support, coping style (especially catastrophic reaction and emotionalism), and prestroke history of depression are early predictors of poststroke depression.

5. Any competent adult has the right to refuse treatment, and if the patient lacks capacity, you need to defer to the closest family members. Explore alternatives, including clerical visits and family involvement, to improve her mood.

BIBLIOGRAPHY

Hollender KD. Screening, diagnosis, and treatment of post-stroke depression. *J Neurosci Nurs.* June 2014;46(3):135–141.
Nabavi SF, Turner A, Dean O, et al. Post-stroke depression therapy: where are we now? *Curr Neurovasc Res.* 2014;11(3):279-289.
Turner A, Hambridge J, White J, et al. Depression screening in stroke: a comparison of alternative measures with the structured diagnostic interview for the diagnostic and statistical manual of mental disorders, fourth edition (major depressive episode) as criterion standard. *Stroke.* April 2012;43(4):1000-1005.

CASE 2: UPPER LIMB PAIN IN STROKE

A 72-year-old male is admitted to the inpatient rehabilitation unit for comprehensive stroke rehabilitation. He has dense right hemiparesis 10 days following the stroke. For the past 2 days he has had right shoulder pain.

Questions

1. Discuss how you would go about evaluating this patient.

2. On physical examination, your patient appears to have pain in the posterior lateral aspect of the shoulder joint. There is a restriction of range of motion due to the pain. The patient has flaccid tone and a 2 fingerbreadth subluxation of the humerus from the glenoid. Discuss management of this patient's shoulder pain.

3. The patient and his family would like to know how subluxation happens and how you would manage it. How are you going to explain this to the family?

4. The patient has completed inpatient rehabilitation and is seeing you in the outpatient clinic 1 month later. His subluxation is now 1 fingerbreadth, but he now has a new burning pain in the shoulder, right hand, and wrist. He has developed some tone in his upper limb, but no significant spasticity. You note swelling, mottled skin, and allodynia. What might be causing this new pain?

5. He returns to your clinic 4 weeks later, and his pain is no better despite physical therapy with mirror therapy, contrast baths, and gentle range of motion. Discuss the treatment of complex regional pain syndrome (CRPS) in stroke.

6. Gabapentin and prednisone have been largely ineffective in controlling his pain, and a stellate ganglion block did not help either. You are considering starting oxycodone in the short term to allow the patient to better participate in his physical therapy. What are considerations in doing this?

CASE 2: UPPER LIMB PAIN IN STROKE

Answers

1. As part of history taking, the patient needs to be asked how the pain began, its quality and severity, and if there are exacerbating and relieving factors. The treating physician needs to know whether the patient had a previous injury or trauma to that shoulder joint, or if there was pre-existing arthritic type shoulder pain. The history taking should focus on possible previous rotator cuff injuries as well. On examination, one has to look for a positive Neer's test, worse shoulder pain with the hand behind the neck maneuver, restriction in passive external rotation at the shoulder joint, evidence of flaccidity versus spasticity, shoulder impingement syndrome, or restriction in range of motion due to pain or weakness. Also look for evidence of subluxation of the shoulder.

2. Management should start with careful positioning of the shoulder to minimize subluxation. This could include a sling if there is significant flaccidity in the upper extremity, and adhesive taping across the shoulder joint. The therapist can provide gentle range of motion exercises. If the patient does not have any contraindications, you can use local analgesic creams and nonsteroidal anti-inflammatories. Many studies have shown improvement in subluxation with therapeutic electrical stimulation, while in other studies there was no significant difference.

3. One has to explain the situation in lay terms. Diagrams are helpful. Shoulder subluxation is characterized by a palpable gap between the acromion and humeral head. During the flaccid period of stroke, the rotator cuff sleeve is not able to maintain the humeral head in the glenoid, and the scapula is downward rotated, predisposing to subluxation. Improper positioning in bed, lack of support when upright, or pulling on the arm during transfers can cause subluxation.

4. The patient probably meets the International Association for Study of Pain (IASP) criteria for CRPS type 1. CRPS type 1 occurs in about 25% of hemiplegic patients with associated spasticity of the involved upper extremity. Lesions of the pre-motor area of the brain especially are associated with CRPS; its etiology still remains unknown. It presents initially with pain in the shoulder followed by painful movements of the wrist and hand. There is hypersensitivity to touch and stiffness of the joints/decreased range of motion, with painful flexion of the wrist and joints of the hand. The pain and edema subside spontaneously in the vast majority of patients in a few weeks.

5. Treatment of CRPS in stroke is controversial and the scientific evidence is sparse. CRPS can be treated with short courses of steroids, such as prednisone, based on small case series and trials. This appears to have better effect when given early in the course, before 13 weeks from onset. Though the mechanism of action is not known, calcitonin intranasally and clodronate and alendronate have been shown to reduce the pain of CRPS. Gabapentin has been shown to be effective in type I CRPS in a randomized, double-blind, placebo-controlled trial. There are no good studies to support use of NSAIDs

and opioids, but they can be tried as an adjunctive treatment. Modalities such as to heat and cold, hand desensitization, and/or mirror therapy may be beneficial. If persistent, stellate ganglion sympathetic block can be considered. The last resort is sympathectomy, with best effect if done within 12 months of onset. To prevent it from getting worse, therapists have to avoid aggressive therapy and carefully position the shoulder with support. The course of CRPS is variable even with treatment, and it may persist for many years.

6. You should screen the patient for risk factors for substance abuse. Ensure that the family will lock up his medications. The most common reason for emergency visits from opioid overdose is family members using a patient's medication. Have them sign an opioid use agreement, which indicates only one physician can prescribe the medication and prohibits early refills. Perform a drug screen before starting. Many practitioners prescribe a dose of naloxone rescue medicine along with the opioid prescription to prevent overdose.

BIBLIOGRAPHY

Cacchio A, De Blasis E, Necozione S, et al. Mirror therapy in complex regional pain syndrome type I of the upper limb in stroke patients. *N Engl J Med.* August 6, 2009;361(6):634-636.

Freedman M, Greis AC, Marino L, et al. Complex regional pain syndrome: diagnosis and treatment. *Phys Med Rehabil Clin N Am.* 2014;25(2):291-303.

CASE 3: DYSPHAGIA

A 72-year-old male is admitted in the inpatient rehabilitation unit with left-sided hemiparesis and cognitive slowing. He had a past medical history of hypertension and hypercholesterolemia and has been placed on medications for secondary stroke prevention. Your nurse indicates that the patient has low-grade fever of 99.6° F with mild tachycardia, and was seen to cough while having his breakfast.

Questions

1. How will you go about evaluating this patient?

2. The speech therapist recommended a modified barium swallow study after the bedside swallow test, and has found the patient has oropharyngeal dysphagia. What are the factors that predispose a stroke patient to aspirate?

3. Your patient's family asks you about the prevalence of dysphagia and the risks associated with dysphagia of acute stroke. Discuss the advice you would give the patient and his family.

4. The resident physician working with you asks what strategies are included in the management of dysphagia. Discuss the best practice guidelines in dysphagia management.

5. What is the current understanding of the benefit of transcutaneous electrical stimulation in the treatment of dysphagia?

CASE 3: DYSPHAGIA

Answers

1. Fever in the stroke patient may be from atelectasis, urinary tract infection, or pneumonia in the acute rehabilitation time frame. While instituting incentive spirometry, the physiatrist has to order a urinalysis and be vigilant for symptoms and signs of an aspiration pneumonia. This is especially true if the patient has evidence of dysphagia. If the stroke patient has productive cough and labs show leukocytosis, a chest x-ray is indicated. As part of the initial evaluation of the stroke, it is a Joint Commission Standard for stroke patients and best practice to get a swallow screen prior to any oral intake such as food, fluid, or medications. You can ask for a speech therapy consultation as part of the evaluation to include a bedside swallow test. Cough reflex testing (CRT) along with water swallow test has high sensitivity and specificity to detect dysphagia. The speech therapist will be able to make an assessment whether the patient needs instrumental evaluation; examples are fiberoptic endoscopic examination of swallow (FEES) or videofluoroscopic modified barium swallow (VMBS), with the latter considered the gold standard in the diagnosis of aspiration.

2. The main factors that affect the stroke patient's ability to safely handle secretions and food are severity of the stroke, location of the stroke in the pontine-medullary region, decreased level of consciousness, cognitive deficits, mobility of the stroke patient, and weak voice and cough. Acidity of the aspirate and also poor oral hygiene are seen to increase the risk of aspiration pneumonia. Dysphagia diets, consisting of textured–modified solid foods and partially thickened liquids, may help to reduce the incidence of aspiration pneumonia.

3. Between 29% and 67% of stroke patients have associated dysphagia and half of them will develop aspiration. One study found that 67% of stroke patients aspirate silently, which is defined as "penetration or food below the level of the true vocal cords, without cough or any outward sign of difficulty" (Linden, Siebens 1983). About 37% of patients who aspirate go on to develop a pneumonia. Aspiration can be detected by a congested voice quality, cough during or after swallowing, or a delay in voluntary initiation of the swallow reflex. Dysphagia is also associated with dehydration and consequent hypotension, especially when the stroke patient has to drink only honey- or nectar-thick liquids. Dysphagia can lead to malnutrition. Studies showed that it is associated with increased length of stay during acute hospitalization and increased institutionalization. Administration of medications is especially challenging in a stroke patient with dysphagia.

4. Suspected patients with dysphagia should be maintained NPO until swallowing status is determined. The speech-language pathologist can recommend an appropriate individualized dysphagia program including appropriate diet. The treating team should monitor hydration status closely, since studies showed that patients with texture-modified dysphagia diets received only

43% of the estimated fluid requirements over the first 21 days post stroke while hospitalized. Regular oral care before each meal helps limit buildup of bacteria. A dietitian can help to assess risk factors of poor nutrition and make recommendations to improve compliance also. The stroke patient with dysphagia should be fed from a seated position, at a slow rate of feeding, ensuring that swallow has taken place before offering additional food or liquid. Limited evidence indicates that a chin-down position prevents aspiration in about 50% of patients who are known aspirators. Position the patient comfortably upright for at least 30 minutes after each meal.

5. Electrical stimulation is widely used in the United States as an adjunct to conventional swallow therapy, but there is conflicting evidence that it can improve swallowing function post stroke. While some studies indicate improvement in the functional oral intake scale (FOIS) scores and fewer episodes of aspiration, others show no change in pharyngeal transit time or aspiration severity.

BIBLIOGRAPHY

Kushner DS, Peters K, Eroglu ST, et al. Neuromuscular electrical stimulation efficacy in acute stroke feeding tube-dependent dysphagia during inpatient rehabilitation. *Am J Phys Med Rehabil.* 2013;92:486-495.

Linden P, Siebens AA. Dysphagia: predicting laryngeal penetration. *Arch Phys Med Rehabil.* June 1983;64(6):281-284.

Miller EL, Murray L, Richards L, et al. Comprehensive overview of nursing and interdisciplinary rehabilitation care of the stroke patient: a scientific statement from the American Heart Association. *Stroke.* 2010;41(10):2402-2448.

Abbreviations

ABG	arterial blood gas	BPM	beats per minute
ABI	ankle-brachial index	CASH	cruciform-anterior-spinal-hyperextension orthosis
ABPMR	American Board of Physical Medicine and Rehabilitation		
		CIMT	constraint-induced movement therapy
ABS Scale	Agitated Behavioral Scale	CMAP	compound motor action potential
ACGME	Accreditation Committee for Graduate Medical Education	COPD	chronic obstructive pulmonary disease
		CPAP	continuous positive airway pressure
ACL	anterior cruciate ligament	CPET	cardiopulmonary exercise test
ADM	abductor digiti minimi		
AFO	ankle foot orthosis	CPK	creatine phosphokinase
AITFL	anterior inferior tibiofibular ligament	CRPS	complex regional pain syndrome
ALS	amyotrophic lateral sclerosis; also known as Lou Gehrig's disease	CRS-R	Coma Recovery Scale-Revised
		CRT	cough reflex testing
ANA	antinuclear antibodies	CSF	cerebrospinal fluid
AP	anteroposterior	CTE	chronic traumatic encephalopathy
APB	abductor pollicis brevis		
ASIS	anterior superior iliac spine	DMII	diabetes mellitus Type 2
AVN	avascular necrosis	EDB	extensor digiti brevis
BDI	Beck Depression Inventory	EF	ejection fraction
		EMG	electromyogram
BiPAP	bilevel positive airway pressure	EMG/NCS	electromyography/ nerve conduction study
BLE	bilateral lower extremities	ESR	erythrocyte sedimentation rate
BMI	body mass index	FABER	flexion, abduction, and external rotation
BMP	basic metabolic panel		

FADIR	flexion, adduction, internal rotation
FDI	first dorsal interosseus
FEES	fiberoptic endoscopic examination of swallow
FM	fibromyalgia
FOIS	functional oral intake scale
FPL	flexor pollicis longus
GDS	Geriatric Depression Scale
GOAT	Galveston Orientation and Amnesia Test
HAART	highly active antiretroviral therapy
HADS	Hospital Anxiety and Depression Scale
HBI	hypoxic brain injury
HIPAA	Health Insurance Portability and Accountability Act
IASP	International Association for Study of Pain
ISNCSCI	International Standards for Neurological Classification of Spinal Cord Injury
IVIG	intravenous immunoglobulin
K-level	a patient's "functional level" for a prosthesis as defined by Medicare
LAD	left anterior descending
LDL	low density lipoprotein
LSO	lumbosacral orthosis
LVEF	left ventricular ejection fraction
MDSBC	Multidisciplinary Spina Bifida Clinic
METs	metabolic equivalents
MI	myocardial infarction
MMA	methylmalonic acid
MMSE	Mini-Mental Status Examination
MOC	maintenance of certification
MoCA	Montreal Cognitive Assessment
MS	multiple sclerosis
MTSS	medial tibial stress syndrome/; also known as shin splints
MUPs	medically unexplained physical symptoms
NCS	nerve conduction studies
NPO	nothing by mouth; latin: nil per os
NSAID	nonsteroidal anti-inflammatory drug
NSE	neuron-specific enolase
OASS	Overt Agitation Severity Scale
OBS	Overt Behaviour Scale
O-log	Orientation-log
PA	posterioanterior
PDQRS	Post-stroke Depression Rating Scale
PDSA	plan, do, see, act
PEG	percutaneous endoscopically placed gastrostomy
PM&R	physical medicine and rehabilitation
PSD	post-stroke depression
PTA	posttraumatic amnesia
PVD	peripheral vascular disease

QI	quality improvement	SPEP	serum protein electrophoresis
RFA	radiofrequency ablation		
RICE	rest, ice, compression, elevation	SSRIs	selective serotonin reuptake inhibitors
ROS	review of systems	SVG	saphenous vein graft
SADQ-H 10/ SADQ-H 21	Stroke Aphasia Depression Questionnaire	TCAs	tricyclic antidepressants
		VAMS	Visual Analog Mood Scale
SI	sacroiliac		
SNRIs	serotonin-norepinephrine reuptake inhibitors	VMBS	videofluoroscopic modified barium swallow
SOMI	sternal occipital mandibular immobilizer	VO_2	oxygen uptake or consumption
SPECT scan	single photon emission computed tomography	VP	ventriculoperitoneal

Index